FAT
LAND

FAT
LAND

....

*How Americans
Became the Fattest People
in the World*

....

Greg Critser

Houghton Mifflin Company

BOSTON   NEW YORK

To my wife, Antoinette Mongelli

For information about permission to reproduce selections from
this book, write to Permissions, Houghton Mifflin Company,
215 Park Avenue South, New York, New York 10003.

Visit our Web site: www.houghtonmifflinbooks.com.

Library of Congress Cataloging-in-Publication Data
Critser, Greg.
Fat land : how Americans became the fattest
people in the world / Greg Critser.
p.   cm.
Includes index.
ISBN 0-618-16472-3
1. Obesity—United States. I. Title.
RA645.O23 C75 2003
362.1'96398'00973—dc21   2002032282

Printed in the United States of America

Book design by Robert Overholtzer

QUM 10 9 8 7 6 5 4 3 2

CONTENTS

ACKNOWLEDGMENTS

This book would not have been possible without the knowledge, wisdom, and generosity of many dedicated individuals, chief among whom were Colin Harrison, my editor at *Harper's,* and Deanne Urmy, my editor at Houghton Mifflin. It was Colin Harrison who first prodded me to write seriously about the subject of obesity, and who held me accountable to the highest standards of journalism in the process. Likewise did Deanne Urmy help me to see the worth in a book-length treatment of the subject. I am also indebted to her for her wit, insight, and passion, which made the path to publication a pleasurable one.

In the process of reporting the many-sided aspects of obesity, I was mentored by two of the best in their respective fields. Professor James O. Hill, of the University of Colorado, was a gentle but tough-minded Virgil in the purgatory of modern epidemiological statistics. Dr. Francine Ratner Kaufman, chief of endocrinology at Children's Hospital Los Angeles and president of the American Diabetes Association, helped me see the real-world implications of obesity statistics and showed me that something can be done about it if one is energetic, compassionate, and tenacious enough. Fortunately for the children of Los Angeles, she is.

A number of other medical and health specialists, all noted in the introductory remarks for each chapter in this book's notes, were of enormous help. A few deserve special recognition. John Peters, Ph.D., of Procter & Gamble's Nutrition Science Institute, provided enlightened and probing comments on the nature of consumerism, consumption, and obesity. Betty Hennessy, of the Los Angeles Office of Education, was a font of information and contacts in the world of physical education. Ash Hayes, the former director of the President's Council on Physical Fitness and

Sports, and Charles Corbin, professor of exercise physiology at the University of Arizona, gave freely of their time answering my many inquiries on the subject of fitness testing. The staff of the USDA's Center for Nutrition Policy and Promotion was critical in obtaining much-needed documents and reports, as was the staff of the National Archives in College Park, Maryland. Finding many obscure journal articles would have been impossible without the reference desk at the Louise M. Darling Biomedical Library at the University of California, Los Angeles. Personal access to scholars was greatly aided by Dunn Gifford and Sara Baer-Sinnott, of Oldways Preservation Trust.

Along the way, a number of friends, teachers, fellow journalists, authors, and editors have also given invaluable support, advice, and criticism. Among them are Joyce Appleby, Michael Balter, Dr. Scott Connelly, Daniel Fineman, Ted Fishman, Eva Fleming, Norris Hundley, Joel Kotkin, Lewis Lapham, Robert Lerner, Stephanie Mencimer, Jeremy Newman, Steve Oney, Richard Rodriguez, Barbara J. Rolls, Mark Salzman, Barry Sanders, Catherine Seipp, Jim Stillwell, and Jessica Yu. Sue Horton published my first personal account of weight loss while an editor at the *LA Weekly,* then made room for several columns on the subject at the *Los Angeles Times,* where she edits the Sunday Opinion section. Dan Ferrara, my editor at *Worth,* carved out space for a remarkable ten thousand–word essay on the subject at that magazine. Glenn Nishimura, my editor at *USA Today,* was a crucial advocate for several op-ed pieces that appeared in those pages.

Special gratitude goes to my agent, Kris Dahl at ICM, for her agile representation, for her cool-headedness, and for always returning my calls.

My family, both nuclear and extended, deserve the lion's share of credit for their unflagging support of my writing career in general, and this book in particular. My mother, Betty Critser, kept me upbeat when things looked dim, as did my sisters, Barbara and Linda, and I am lucky to have inherited the work ethic of my late father, Paul C. Critser. My culinary mentor and mother-in-law, Julia Mongelli, kept me rooted to reality in matters of food and food politics. Nicholas and Christopher Coauette and Elliott Haberman likewise provided a reality check on what children really want to eat (which is, from what I can gather, candy . . . *now!*). A huge thanks — and *grazie!* — goes as well to the Spence, Stromei, Caiolfi, Lanaghan, Raguseo, and Macchia families.

This book is dedicated to my wife, Antoinette Mongelli, who was a constant source of inspiration, support, good will, insight, humor, joy, and love. Without her, *Fat Land* would still be between my ears.

INTRODUCTION

Obesity is the dominant unmet global health issue,
with Western countries topping the list.

— World Health Organization

Set the soul of thy son aright, and all the rest will
be added hereafter!

— Saint John Chrysostom

THIS BOOK is not a memoir, but it is undeniably grounded in a
singular personal experience. My experience was not, for those
hoping for something juicy, a moment of childhood drama. Nor
was it anything that led to any form of spiritual or true psychological revelation. Compared to the harrowing tribulations that so
much of the world's population endures, it was, when all is said
and done, rather mundane and petty. Here it is: Some guy called
me fatso. Specifically, he screamed: "Watch it, fatso!"

Here I should note that I deserved the abuse; after all, I had
opened my car door into a busy street without looking into my
side mirror first, and so had nearly decapitated the poor fellow. I
could have killed him. But why . . . *fatso?* Could it be because I
was indeed forty pounds overweight? Or that I could not fit into

any of my clothes, even the ones I got at the Gap that were labeled "relaxed" (which, come to think of it, I wasn't), let alone the ones considered "baggy" (which, again come to think of it, I was)? Could it be because I had to back up ten feet so as to get my entire face into the bathroom mirror to shave every morning? Or that when I dined with friends they hid their small pets and seemed to guard their plates, one arm curled around them, as if I might plunge my fork into their juicy pieces of duck and make off with them? I'm obviously joking about the latter, but the point is that the insult hit home. In upwardly mobile, professional America, being fat — and having someone actually notice it and say something about it — is almost as bad as getting caught reading *Playboy* in your parents' bedroom when you're ten. Shame shame shame.

Fatness was hardly a new issue for me. My wife and my physician had been after me for some time to do something about my problem, the former quite gingerly, the latter not so. My doctor, in fact, had recently suggested that I consider a new weight loss medication. At the time, I had promptly brushed the idea aside. Now, the sting still fresh, I reconsidered: Why not?

And so, for the next nine months, I put all of my extra energy into the task of shedding my excess avoirdupois. In modern America, this, I would find, was a rite in itself, replete with its own social institutions (health clubs), tonics (Meridia), taboos (Krispy Kreme), and aspirational totems (Levi's 501 regular cuts). I was apparently ready for this rite, for, to my delight, I slowly but surely lost the weight. What followed was encouraging, if somewhat predictable: congratulations from friends for "sticking to it"; enhanced self-esteem; a new wardrobe; a newfound confidence and spring in my step; phone calls from J.Lo. and Julia.

Yet the more I contemplated my success, the more I came to see it not as a triumph of will, but as a triumph of my economic and social class. The weight loss medication Meridia, for example, had been effective not because it is such a good drug; even its purveyors freely admit it is far from effective for most people. What had made the drug work for me was the upper-middle-class support system that I had brought to it: a good physician who insisted on seeing me every two weeks, access to a safe park where I would walk and jog, friends who shared the value of becoming slender, healthy home-cooked food consumed with my wife, books about health, and medical journals about the latest nutritional breakthroughs. And money. And time.

I wrote about these insights, first for a local magazine, then in my column in *USA Today,* where I write about the politics of health. I then moved on to other topics. As is the case with most subject matter, fatness had remained, at least for me, somewhat abstract, distant — intellectual rather than emotional. It was certainly nothing one could view as a matter of national urgency.

Then, two things happened which would change that.

For one, I met a man named James O. Hill. Hill is a physiologist at the University of Colorado's Health Sciences Center. Curly-haired, a bit provocative, Hill is a vigorous, intellectually engaged fellow with an agile debating style and a wide-ranging presence in his field. Hill's field is the study of obesity, everything from its epidemiology to its causes to its treatment. It was Hill who, only a few years ago, coined what may be the single most quoted line in regard to today's soaring obesity rates. "If obesity is left unchecked," he told the Associated Press, "almost all Americans will be overweight by 2050." Becoming obese, he went on, "is a normal response to the American environment." With a presence on all of the leading public health committees charged with doing something about the nation's expanding waistline, Hill is the dean of obesity studies. It was my fortune to meet him at just the right time.

Hill spelled out the problem more clearly than anyone else. "See, for decades, most of us believed that the rate of overweight in this country was relatively static — somewhere around 25 percent of the population would be always overweight," he recalled one day. "But then, beginning in the late eighties, we started see-

3

ing that rate spike upward, 30, 35, 40 percent. And that started freaking a lot of us out. Where were the gains coming from? We know that obesity has a strong genetic component, but twenty years — anyone knows that is a laughingly small amount of time for genetics to change so much. So for the guys like myself, the question has become, basically, what has changed in the environment to allow the inclination toward overweight and obesity to express itself? What changed around us to allow us to get so big?"

Main Question

Big, of course, is putting it mildly. Today Americans are the fattest people on the face of the earth (save for the inhabitants of a few South Seas islands). About 61 percent of Americans are overweight — overweight enough to begin experiencing health problems as a direct result of that weight. About 20 percent of us are obese — so fat that our lives will likely be cut short by excess fat. More than 5 million Americans now meet the definition of morbid obesity; they are so obese that they qualify for a radical surgical technique known as gastroplasty, wherein the stomach is surgically altered so as to keep food from being digested. (The American Bariatric Society, whose members perform gastroplasty, reports that its waiting lists are months long and that its surgeons "can't keep up.")

Children are most at risk from obesity. About 25 percent of all Americans under age nineteen are overweight or obese, a figure that, Hill points out, has doubled in thirty years. That one figure recently moved U.S. Surgeon General Dr. David Satcher to declare obesity to be a national epidemic. "Today," he told a group of federal bureaucrats and health policy officers, "we see a nation of young people seriously at risk of starting out obese and dooming themselves to the difficult task of overcoming a tough illness."

Obesity itself is slowly moving into the middle and upper classes, but the condition disproportionately plagues the poor and the working poor. Mexican American women aged 20 to 74, for example, have an obesity rate about 13 percent higher for those living below the poverty line versus those above the poverty line. Diabetes occurs at a rate of 16 to 26 percent in both Hispanic and black Americans aged 45 to 74, compared to 12 percent in non-Hispanic whites of the same age.

Yet most of America — particularly the America of the Me Generation — seems to be in deep denial about the class and age aspects of obesity. Get a group of boomers together and, within minutes, the topic of obesity shifts not to medical issues but, rather, to aesthetic and gender issues, to the notion — widely held in the urban upper middle class — that "talking too much about obesity just ends up making kids have low self-esteem." Or that it "might lead to anorexia."

Those attitudes also permeate the medical sphere; doctors and other health care providers remain either in ignorance or outright denial about the health danger to the poor and the young. In a rare moment of industry scrutiny a few years ago, the Centers for Disease Control surveyed twelve thousand obese adults to find out what, exactly, their doctors were telling them. The results were arresting. Fewer than half reported being advised to lose weight. A separate study sharpened the indictment: Patients with incomes above $50,000 were more likely to receive such advice than were those with incomes below. As the *Journal of the American Medical Association* noted, "The lower rates of counseling among respondents with lower education and income levels . . . are particularly worrisome, because members of lower socioeconomic groups have poorer health outcomes."

Yes, worrisome. Yet we Americans are inured to such dirges, which daily seem to well up from the pages of our newspapers. Certainly I was. Until, that is, the unexpected intruded.

It happened in the Intensive Care Unit of Los Angeles County/ USC Medical Center, one of the nation's busiest hospitals. I was there visiting an ailing relative when, suddenly, a gaggle of interns, nurses, and orderlies pushed a gurney through the ward. On it lay a very large young man, perhaps 450 pounds, hooked to the ganglia of modern medicine. He had just undergone an emergency gastroplasty repair, and it did not look good. As I came to learn, first through bits and pieces exchanged by the ward nurses, then through comments by the patient's parents, it was not the first emergency for this man. As his mother, a modestly dressed woman in her forties, moaned at one point, "Second time in three months . . . his stomach keeps coming unstapled" (not all forms of gastroplasty actually involve stapling, as did older forms of obesity surgery, but many still refer to it that way). The woman then leaned on the shoulder of her weary husband. "My . . . boy." Her boy was dying from his own fat.

Yes, he was dying, and yes, the more I looked, the more I could see: Here was someone's boy, one plagued, I imagined, by years of bad health, discomfort, self-loathing, and, of course, countless insults and snickers by passersby and friends alike. But someone's little boy nonetheless. Watching him as he gasped for air — respiratory function is one of the first things that can go when one gets so big — I could not help think: There but for the grace of God go I. And, to hear Jim Hill and Dr. Satcher tell it, a large number of other decent Americans.

Driving home that night, through the barrio of East L.A., then up the chilly black Pasadena Freeway to the town where I live, I wondered just how a boy becomes so disabled. Genes certainly played a role, but as Jim Hill had lucidly pointed out, genes have always played a role in obesity. The question was, why are we seeing so many more people like the one I just saw? How — exactly — had they been made? And if it is true that, in America, every man is his own author, that every man, as Ivan Illich once wrote, "is responsible for what has been made of him," then what, as a nation, is being made of us by the obese?

I decided to find out: How is it that we better-off Americans, perhaps the most health-conscious of any generation in the history of the world, have come to preside over the deadly fattening of our youth and their future? That is the story you will read on the following pages, and that is why we must now turn to the strange career of one Earl L. Butz . . .

1

UP UP UP!

(*Or, Where the Calories Came From*)

EARL BUTZ, nominated by Richard Nixon in 1971 to be the eighteenth secretary of agriculture, conjured the airs of a courtly midwestern grandfather, the kind who liked to show up at Sunday dinner, give the blessing, lecture the grandchildren about patriotism, free trade, the goodness of farm life, and the evils that threatened such a life — and then go out to the backyard and tell off-color jokes to the assembled adults.

In Washington, Butz was an optimist, chanting "Up up up!" whenever he got good news about farm prices. And he was telegenic, his hawk-nosed profile and slicked-back white hair a staple on the nightly news, where he would spin his own "up up up" version of America and its endless agricultural cornucopia. Indeed, if most Nixon appointees avoided the light and the heat, Butz bathed in it. There were his endless battles with Henry Kissinger, whom Butz liked to accuse of "putting your dirty fingers into my farm policy." There was his constant — and very public — denigration of welfare spending, of people who "sit on their duff waiting for a nice handout." And there was his persona in his office, where Butz would regale visitors with his grand visions for agriculture — better crops! tastier tomatoes! corn and wheat and rice to feed a hungry world! — and then, grinning like a Rockwellian Puck, jerk his thumb backward at the sculpture sitting behind his desk — one of two wooden elephants, copulating. "That's what it was like trying to multiply the farm vote for Nixon!" he'd say with an infectious belly laugh. It was hard not to conclude that Earl "Rusty" Butz was, among many other things, a true piece of work.

Like most presidents, Richard Nixon had nominated his new agriculture secretary for largely political reasons. By the early 1970s the once solid "farm vote" was wobbling. The problem was the economy; farm income had plummeted. The immediate causes were short term in nature. Cautious growers simply had not planted enough grain crops. At the same time, the costs of farming — from agrochemicals to labor to transportation — had soared, so much so that by 1972 poultry farmers were forced to kill a million baby chicks because they could not afford the price of feed. Urbanization drove the long-term forces behind the farm problem. Cropland was getting more and more expensive to hold on to. So was labor. Old-timers were seeing their grandchildren go off to college — and not return. Anyone with political antennae could see that the overall mood was one of gloom — not a particularly promising mood for what many believed would be a hotly contested election. When profits hit an all-time low in 1971, farm leaders began openly talking about defecting to the Democrats. Nixon, preoccupied with the Vietnam War and dogged by the press, despaired: A bunch of angry farmers was all he needed.

But the president did know one thing: To fix the farm, he needed someone from the farm. And in 1971, Butz — conservative, energetic, with an already lengthy vita ranging from his Ph.D. in agricultural economics to his service to the United Nation's Food and Agricultural Organization — was a perfect farm fixer.

Not long after Butz arrived in Washington, though, another crisis exploded, this one involving a character as truculent as Butz himself: the American consumer. Around the nation, homemakers were fuming at the soaring prices of such basic items as hamburger, cheese, sugar — even margarine. By early 1973, with food price inflation at an all-time high, the anger had turned into a full-blown middle-class protest. Across the country, consumer groups comprising self-described activist homemakers organized a widespread meat boycott, replete with big-city marches and signs that read HELP US HELP YOU! DON'T EAT MEAT! The movement even had its own graphics — a big T-bone steak with BOYCOTT MEAT emblazoned across it in giant red letters. In San Francisco, the Consumer Action Group called for a 15 percent price rollback for all meat. (Nixon responded with a poorly received "price ceiling.") In Houston, Housewives for Collective Action led their entire families on loud demonstrations at supermarkets. The July 16 issue of *U.S. News & World Report* summed up the national discontent perfectly: "Why a food scare in a land of plenty?"

The answer was meteorological and global. The weather in 1972 had been abnormally bad for farmers worldwide, resulting in smaller crops across the board. Worse, a basic source of protein feed meal for the world, the anchovy fisheries off the coast of Peru, failed to produce even minimal requirements. Add to this the impact of the devalued dollar, which made American food cheaper abroad just as supplies were dropping worldwide. The result was that there wasn't enough food — or at least not enough food to keep prices stable. Around the country, the situation provoked rampant malaise-speak, even among typically cool-headed observers. "Like it or not," declared the economist Lester R. Brown of the Overseas Development Council, "Americans are sharing food scarcity with Russia." Suddenly, there were signs of shortage fear everywhere. Stores selling horse meat opened in Portland and Chicago. In Minnesota, a black market in meat was reported.

To Nixon, the political face of food had warped. If farmers wanted more money for their products, consumers wanted products for less money. With notions of entitlement growing and memories of the Depression fading, the folks "wanted what they wanted when they wanted it," as Butz liked to put it. And Butz, disinclined to equivocation — "The only one thing in the middle of the road is a dead skunk!" — was inclined to please the farmers first.

To do so he launched an aggressive campaign to "liberate" growers from the clutch of government regulation. To enlarge the farmer's marketplace, he spiked USDA rules requiring government approval for large export sales. In late 1973 he went abroad to beat down trade barriers to American products, later striking the nation's largest grain sale ever to a foreign power, the Soviet Union. And to give the farmer more pricing flexibility, he ended the longtime program of mandated national grain siloing, instead letting farmers store and sell excess grain where and when they desired. His message caught on. Corn and soybean growers planted their fields exactly as the Sage of Purdue advised: "from fencerow to fencerow." By the mid-1970s corn production soared to an all-time high. So did farm income.

For makers of convenience foods, the corn surpluses would eventually become a boon to new product development and sales. For years, sugar prices had been tied to a worldwide price structure that, in essence, served as a form of foreign aid to developing nations. That had kept prices for U.S. consumers — manufacturers and families alike — unnaturally high. But in 1971 food scientists in Japan found a way to economically produce a cheaper sweetener. They called it high-fructose corn syrup, or HFCS. It was six times sweeter than cane sugar and, as its name implied, it could be made from corn. That meant that the cost of producing any high-sugar product could be slashed. HFCS had other chemical attributes as well. Using it in frozen foods protected the product against freezer burn. Using it in long-shelf-life products — like those in vending machines — kept the product fresh-tasting. Using it in bakery products (even in rolls and biscuits that normally contained no sugar) made those products look "more natural" — as if they had just been browned in the oven. Although it would not be until the late 1970s that mass production techniques would make its use widespread, HFCS stood as a testimony to Butz's free-planting theology.

HFCS also had one attribute that posed a potentially troubling question to those in the food industry. Fructose, unlike sucrose or dextrose, took a decidedly different route into the human metabolism. Where the latter would go through a complex breakdown process before arriving in the human liver, the former, for some reason, bypassed that breakdown and arrived almost completely intact in the liver, whereupon the organ set upon it as it would anything else. This unique feature of fructose, which was intensified by the high concentrations of it in HFCS, would come to be called "metabolic shunting." In food science circles, it raised eyebrows but, as several scientists present at the time note, not warning flags. Stanley Segall, now a leading expert in the science of fat and sugar replacements at Drexel University in Philadelphia, recalls a committee he served on at the time that was looking at the fructose shunting issue. "I remember being told, as a sort of junior on the committee, 'Don't be silly — everyone knows that it's the same as sugar.' But no one really answered the question: whether, if you use fructose as your main source of sweetener, you *do* get more fructose in the metabolic process," he says today. "It was decided fructose was no different — that it was only a question of quantity. But no one really looked at it in depth."

Certainly not the USDA. There the concern was pure farm economics. To stimulate demand for his farmers' goods, Butz took to the stump to "re-educate" the caterwauling American consumer. Striding up onto a makeshift platform in a supermarket parking lot, Butz would pull a loaf of Wonder Bread from a paper bag and wave it about for all to see. "You all know what this is," he'd say, opening the bag and pulling out a single slice. "Well, guess how much is the farmer's share of this. You'd be right if you said this one darned slice!"

Consumers had the problem all wrong, Butz would go on.

Why, it was the labor unions — particularly the transport, manufacturing, and retail sectors — that caused the greatest price increases. Their average wage increases had gone up while the farmer's typical wages had stayed flat. Labor leaders like George Meany were the problem. The supermarket barons were the problem. Even consumers bore some of the responsibility. Convenience foods and TV dinners (still costly then) were really nothing but a "built-in maid service." The meat boycott wasn't the answer. Everyone needed simply to buck up.

But the straight talk that had worked with farmers wasn't enough for American consumers. Many of them were union members themselves, struggling just to make ends meet. Others were members of a new kind of American family, one consisting of not one but two wage earners. To them TV dinners might be pricey, but they were also practical. And wanting meat every day was not a bad thing. A cartoon in the *New York Times Magazine* depicting a man and his wife sitting down to table with two bowls of dog food caught the mood. Holding back Rover with one hand and holding out a newspaper with the other, the man reads: "Secretary Butz says the price of steak is just right!"

Of course it wasn't. And the consumer message to Washington — a veritable generational temper tantrum — was clear: We want what we want when we want it. We don't care why food is expensive, we just want it to be less so. You're the government — fix it, or we'll turn you out in October. Richard Nixon, of course, was gone long before then.

Gerald Ford, the reluctant new president, was a quiet, deliberate man with the impossible task of reassuring "the folks" that a post-Nixon government of Republicans could be trusted. He was, like the nation, obsessed with inflation, and in his office and on the stump he liked to refer to the problem as "public enemy number one." To squash the enemy he turned to Butz. His only instructions were to get food prices down without resorting to the kind of price controls that Nixon had implemented in 1973.

One day, pondering this new charge, Butz got a phone call

from a Texas congressman named William Poage. The assistant chair of the influential House Committee on Agriculture, Poage was often on the horn to Butz, usually complaining about this import subsidy or that export restriction — anything that might damage his powerful constituency of soybean growers. He certainly never called to praise the secretary, who had alone championed the opening of overseas markets for Poage's bean growers — markets that, almost overnight, had made them the single richest agricultural producers in the world.

"Mr. Secretary — it's rat oil," Poage said in his dry Texas drawl.

"What?"

"It's rat oil, sir. This palm oil thing has gotten completely out of hand. We've got to do something. We can't just sit here and let the Malays take our markets away from . . ."

Butz had been getting updates about a congressional debate over the issue of palm oil imports and its impact on soybean growers. As usual with Poage, the soybean growers faced "a national crisis." They were at "a dangerous turning point." The secretary, Poage complained, had told the nation's farmers to plant fencerow to fencerow. Now where were they going to sell all those soybeans if we were going to allow this "rat oil" — Poage was convinced, albeit without any evidence, that it was "infested" — to take away our own home markets?

The congressman went on and on, but to Butz his plaint — and the message from much of his own constituency — had grown predictable and confounding, especially in light of the president's new mandate. Poage wanted the administration to back new quotas and tariffs on Malaysian palm oil. Butz was chagrined. As he recalled in a recent interview, "It was back to square one with the education campaign. The hardest thing to sell — and get the American farmer to understand — was that to expand exports we had to expand imports. We had to get farmers to think differently. They had been used to being protected. Yet the president wanted the government out of the farming business.

"So what was I to do?" Butz continued. "I finally came to the

13

conclusion that I would have to take some heat to get the point across — even if it was from our own constituency." The new official line, Butz explained, was "to stand up for free trade on both sides — it was the only way I was going to keep some legitimacy bringing down other barriers abroad. President Ford gave me a lot more freedom than President Nixon, so I was able to go ahead on something that should have been done a long time ago."

Freed from Kissinger's "dirty little fingers" in international matters, Butz moved his new agenda quickly. To delay any new tariff or import legislation, he deployed his closest political staff to testify in front of a House Agriculture Committee meeting, where Poage was in high boil. Butz instructed his staff to tell the representatives that he would have to prepare a special report before considering their demands, and that the report would not be ready until May. The stall thus lodged, Butz assembled a group of his most ardent free trade advisers and planned what they came to call "the round the world free trade mission." Palm oil would be one of its first subjects, and Malaysia, where the bulk of it was grown and processed, would be one of his mission's first stops.

Palm oil had been around as a commercial fat for many years. The British had introduced *Elaeis guineensis* as a plantation crop in the late nineteenth century. Later on, the Malaysian government had subsidized the palm's widespread planting as a way to resettle thousands of poor Malays onto the new nation's rugged frontier. But palm oil, which is more chemically similar to beef tallow than traditional vegetable oil, was difficult to process. Some of its original American importers referred to it as axle grease. Its competitors called it tree lard.

In the mid-1970s, however, new technologies transformed tree lard into a viable commercial fat, one fit for everything from frying french fries to making margarine to baking cookies and bread and pies and no end of convenience ("built-in maid service") foods. It was, in a sense, the fat world's compatriot to the sugar world's HFCS. Because it was a stable fat, products made with *palm oil* it lasted forever on supermarket shelves. True, a manufacturer might have to use more of it to achieve a good "mouthfeel," and that meant an increased caloric count in the resultant food product, but that, at least at the time, was a secondary issue. Price was key. And palm oil prices were unbelievably good — all the time. The trees produced heavily all year round. Palm oil was also tastier than many vegetable oils, mainly because of its molecular similarities to lard. There was one other thing: Palm oil was such a highly saturated fat that its proponents secretly touted it as "cow fat disguised as vegetable oil."

American health and medical experts already knew that saturated fats were bad for the cardiovascular system, plugging up arteries, sending blood pressure spiraling, and raising the chances that a consumer of such fats might die a premature death. In the Agriculture Committee's hearings on palm oil, Poage himself tried to marshal the health argument. "Palm oil is more highly saturated than hog lard," he testified. "I do not think that the American housewife should be put to the proposition of buying this palm oil without any notice whatever that it is not what she thinks it is. She thinks when she buys vegetable oil that that's all there is to it, and that she has got something good for her family. When she buys this type of vegetable oil, she ought to have a warning." Hence, in his bill, Poage proposed that all food containing palm oil come with a label stating that it "contains or was prepared or processed with palm oil, a highly saturated imported vegetable product."

Although Poage was more interested in the economic damage that palm oil was wreaking upon his soybean constituency than in its health impacts, he also happened to be on target. Hog lard, even then rarely used, was 38 percent saturated; palm oil was 45 percent saturated. His idea to label palm oil as a saturated fat was ten years ahead of its time. Yet in Congress, not a single medical authority testified against palm oil. As much as the medical establishment was concerned about saturated fats, palm oil seemed an unlikely candidate to be singled out for censure. The small body of science on the fat was mixed. It had been linked to gallstones in hamsters and hypertension in rats. But it also had been assessed positively because of its ability to prevent vitamin A deficiency in such nutritionally underdeveloped nations as Indonesia. Public health advocates were hardly prepared for a battle. The U.S. regulatory system for foods, split between the boosterish USDA and the overburdened FDA, was hardly the place to initiate and fund speculative food science. Then, as now, foods were lightly regulated; their long-term medical consequences were less important than their immediate safety, purity, and usefulness.

And then, as now, food was an increasingly globalized political issue. In Malaysia, palm oil could make or break a career, and Butz's counterpart, Musa bin Hitam, had ridden it to the crest of power. Tough-minded and pragmatic, Hitam ran the country's powerful Ministry of Primary Industries, which among other things was responsible for palm oil production and sales. He operated the ministry like a business, setting goals for his staff and making quick response to trade queries a priority. Americans doing business in Kuala Lumpur knew Hitam as a progressive bureaucrat and a worthy negotiator.

On April 23, 1976, Hitam met Butz at Kuala Lumpur International airport and swept him off to a series of stopovers. The stops were meant to impress one message upon Butz: If Malaysia were to remain a strong ally in a still volatile Southeast Asia, the country needed enhanced trade with the United States and other developed nations. As Hitam later wrote, the palm oil trade was a "fuel for democracy."

"You must realize that 85 to 90 percent of our national budget comes from what I look after," Hitam told Butz. "In rubber alone, each 1 percent increase means $25 million in export earning for us." The same was true with palm oil, Hitam went on. Palm oil wasn't like soybean oil, which was merely a by-product of soy meal production. "It's a big bit of our entire earnings, sir."

As the two men strode through a palm plantation in Selangor, Butz began to warm to Hitam, recalls John DeCourcy, a senior agricultural attaché in the U.S. embassy in Kuala Lumpur at the time. Soon the secretary was telling funny stories from his own repertoire that illustrated the American version of Hitam's concerns.

"And he managed to get Hitam talking about something that no other American ever did: What could America sell to Malaysia?" DeCourcy recalls. "Traditionally all of Malaysia's imports — chicken parts, canned goods, even orange juice — had come from Europe, usually via some U.K. group that had longtime colonial ties. But Mr. Butz — he connected with this guy like no other I'd ever seen. Why, he even sat down and ate durian [one of the most foul-smelling fruits in the world] with him — and without betraying even a hint of discomfort or surprise."

Only two days after the visit, DeCourcy and Hitam both received messages from Butz. To Hitam he wrote: "May I assure you again that we intend to remain competitive in the edible oil field . . . and that means access to our markets. . . . We are delighted with your plans for product diversification, market development, and market diversification. We feel your interest and our interest in this area are identical." To DeCourcy he wrote that "we are going to stand foursquare for the principles of freer trade."

In other words, Poage be damned. Palm oil would be welcomed in America.

Reading his letter and breathing a sigh of relief, DeCourcy couldn't help but chuckle. He had just witnessed a deal that could alter the course of a nation — one that had been pulled off by a quirky man from Purdue who could eat a smelly durian with the relish of a farm boy chomping down on the season's first ripe watermelon.

Earl "Rusty" Butz, of course, would be remembered by most Americans not for his accomplishments in bringing down the cost of food, but rather for his one great vice: joke-telling. His most infamous — and last — official transgression took place in September 1976, when Butz was flying from the GOP convention in Kansas City to Los Angeles with a group of friends. It was late. The secretary was tired. Bored, he began telling jokes. Asked by John Dean why Republicans couldn't get more African Americans into their tent, Butz replied with an anecdote he'd heard from an old ward politician, something to the effect that all blacks really wanted was sex, loose shoes, and indoor plumbing. Dean published the remarks in an article he was writing for *Rolling Stone*. Gerald Ford, in a tight election campaign, castigated Butz. His own party stalwarts urged him to fire Butz. The president refused. The press picked up on the infighting and within a week, Earl Butz had resigned and returned to Purdue.

By the early 1980s, however, Butz's true legacy was everywhere evident. There were no more shortages of meat or butter or sugar or coffee. Prices on just about every single commodity were down, as were the prices of foods made with such commodities. In what would prove to be one of the single most important changes to the nation's food supply, both Coke and Pepsi switched from a fifty-fifty blend of sugar and corn syrup to 100 percent high-fructose corn syrup. The move saved both companies 20 percent in sweetener costs, allowing them to boost portion sizes and still make substantial profits.

Meat production worldwide soared as feed costs of soy meal and corn fell. That, in turn, spurred huge increases in the supply of soybean oil, a by-product, leading to even lower prices for that industrial fat. At the supermarket, calorie-dense convenience foods were thus becoming more and more affordable. High-fructose corn syrup made from the growing surpluses of U.S. corn had made it easier and less expensive to make frozen foods. TV dinners and boxed macaroni and cheese were downright cheap. At fast-food stands, portions were getting bigger. Fries were tasting better and better and getting cheaper and cheaper. (McDonald's, which at that time fried its potatoes in palm oil, had built its first Malaysian oil processing plant just months after Butz's visit.) And the very presence of such alternatives as palm oil forced traditional fat suppliers like the soybean growers to lower their prices as well.

In short, Butz had delivered everything the modern American consumer had wanted. A new plenitude of cheap, abundant, and tasty calories had arrived.

It was time to eat.

2

....

SUPERSIZE ME

(Who Got the Calories into Our Bellies)

I F THE WOBBLY ECONOMY of the 1970s had left consumers fulminating over high food prices and the forces that caused them, the same economy had driven David Wallerstein, a peripatetic director of the McDonald's Corporation, to rage against a force even more primal: cultural mores against gluttony. He hated the fifth deadly sin because it kept people from buying more hamburgers.

Wallerstein had first waged war on the injunction against gluttony as a young executive in the theater business. At the staid Balaban Theaters chain in the early 1960s, Wallerstein had realized that the movie business was really a margin business; it wasn't the sale of low-markup movie tickets that generated profits but rather the sale of high-markup snacks like popcorn and Coke. To sell more of such items, he had, by the mid-1960s, tried about every trick in the conventional retailer's book: two-for-one specials, combo deals, matinee specials, etc. But at the end of any given day, as he tallied up his receipts, Wallerstein inevitably came up with about the same amount of profit.

Thinking about it one night, he had a realization: People did not want to buy two boxes of popcorn *no matter what.* They didn't want to be seen eating two boxes of popcorn. It looked . . . piggish. So Wallerstein flipped the equation around: Perhaps he could get more people to spend just a little more on popcorn if he made the boxes bigger and increased the price only a little. The popcorn cost a pittance anyway, and he'd already paid for the salt and the seasoning and the counter help and the popping machine. So he put up signs advertising jumbo-size popcorn.

The results after the first week were astounding. Not only were individual sales of popcorn increasing; with them rose individual sales of that other high-profit item, Coca-Cola.

Later, at McDonald's in the mid-1970s, Wallerstein faced a similar problem: With consumers watching their pennies, restaurant customers were coming to the Golden Arches less and less frequently. Worse, when they did, they were "cherry-picking," buying only, say, a small Coke and a burger, or, worse, just a burger, which yielded razor-thin profit margins. How could he get people back to buying more fries? His popcorn experience certainly suggested one solution — sell them a jumbo-size bag of the crispy treats.

Yet try as he may, Wallerstein could not convince Ray Kroc, McDonald's founder, to sign on to the idea. As recounted in interviews with his associates and in John F. Love's 1985 book, *McDonald's: Behind the Arches,* the exchange between the two men could be quite contentious on the issue. "If people want more fries," Kroc would say, "they can buy two bags."

"But Ray," Wallerstein would say, "they don't want to eat two bags — they don't want to look like a glutton."

To convince Kroc, Wallerstein decided to do his own survey of customer behavior, and began observing various Chicago-area McDonald's. Sitting in one store after another, sipping his drink and watching hundreds of Chicagoans chomp their way through their little bag of fries, Wallerstein could see: People *wanted* more fries.

"How do you know that?" Kroc asked the next morning when Wallerstein presented his findings.

"Because they're eating the entire bagful, Ray," Wallerstein said. "They even scrape and pinch around at the bottom of the bag for more and eat the salt!"

Kroc gave in. Within months receipts were up, customer counts were up, and franchisees — the often truculent heart and soul of the McDonald's success — were happier than ever.

Many franchisees wanted to take the concept even further, offering large-size versions of other menu items. At this sudden burst of entrepreneurism, however, McDonald's mid-level managers hesitated. Many of them viewed large-sizing as a form of "discounting," with all the negative connotations such a word evoked. In a business where "wholesome" and "dependable" were the primary PR watchwords, large-sizing could become a major image problem. Who knew what the franchisees, with their primal desires and shortcutting ways, would do next? No, large-sizing was something to be controlled tightly from Chicago, if it were to be considered at all.

Yet as McDonald's headquarters would soon find out, large-sizing was a new kind of marketing magic — a magic that could not so easily be put back into those crinkly little-size bags.

Max Cooper, a Birmingham franchisee, was not unfamiliar with marketing and magic; for most of his adult life he had been paid to conjure sales from little more than hot air and smoke. Brash, blunt-spoken, and witty, Cooper had acquired his talents while working as an old-fashioned public relations agent — the kind, as he liked to say, who "got you into the newspaper columns instead of trying to keep you out." In the 1950s with his partner, Al Golin, he had formed what later became Golin Harris, one of the world's more influential public relations firms. In the mid-1960s, first as a consultant and later as an executive, he had helped create many of McDonald's most successful early campaigns. He had been the prime mover in the launch of Ronald McDonald.

By the 1970s Cooper, tired of "selling for someone else," bought a couple of McDonald's franchises in Birmingham, moved his split-off ad agency there, and set up shop as an independent businessman. As he began expanding, he noticed what many other McDonald's operators were noticing: declining customer counts. Sitting around a table and kibitzing with a few like-minded associates one day in 1975, "we started talking about how we could build sales — how we could do it and be profitable," Cooper recalled in a recent interview. "And we realized we could do one of three things. We could cut costs, but there's a limit to that. We could cut prices, but that too has its limits. Then we could raise sales profitably — sales, after all, could be limitless when you think about it. We realized we could do that by taking the high-profit drink and fry and then packaging it with the low-profit burger. We realized that if you could get them to buy three items for what they perceived as less, you could substantially drive up the number of walk-ins. Sales would follow."

But trying to sell that to corporate headquarters was next to impossible. "We were maligned! Oh were we maligned," he recalls. "A 99-cent anything was heresy to them. They would come and say 'You're just cutting prices! What are we gonna look like to everybody else?'"

"No no no," Cooper would shoot back. "You have to think of the analogy to a fine French restaurant. You always pay less for a *table d'hôte* meal than you pay for *à la carte,* don't you?"

"Yes, but —"

"Well, this is a *table d'hôte,* dammit! You're getting more people to the table spending as much as they would before — and coming more often!"

Finally headquarters relented, although by now it hardly mattered. Cooper had by then begun his own rogue campaign. He was selling what the industry would later call "value meals" — the origin of what we now call supersizing. Using local radio, he advertised a "Big Mac and Company," a "Fish, Fry, Drink and Pie," a "4th of July Value Combo."

Sales, Cooper says, "went through the roof. Just like I told them they would."

*   *   *

Selling more for less, of course, was hardly a revolutionary notion, yet in one sense it was, at least to the purveyors of restaurant food in post-Butzian America. Where their prewar counterparts sold individual meals, the profitability of which depended on such things as commodity prices and finicky leisure-time spending, the fast-food vendors of the early 1980s sold a product that obtained its profitability from a consumer who increasingly viewed their product as a necessity. Profitability came by maintaining the total average tab.

The problem with maintaining spending levels was inflation. By the early Reagan years, inflation — mainly through rising labor costs — had driven up the average fast-food tab, causing a decline in the average head count. To bring up the customer count by cutting prices was thus viewed as a grand and — despite the anecdotal successes of people like Wallerstein and Cooper — largely risky strategy. But one thing was different: Thanks to Butz, the baseline costs of meat, bread, sugar, and cheese were rising much more slowly. There was some "give" in the equation if you could somehow combine that slight advantage with increased customer traffic. But how to get them in the door?

In 1983 the Pepsi Corporation was looking for such a solution when it hired John Martin to run its ailing Taco Bell fast-food operation. A Harley-riding, Hawaiian shirt–wearing former Burger King executive, Martin arrived with few attachments to fast-food tradition. "Labor, schmabor!" he liked to say whenever someone sat across from him explaining why, for the millionth time, you couldn't get average restaurant payroll costs down.

But Martin quickly found out that, as Max Cooper had divined a decade before, traditional cost-cutting had its limits. If you focused on it too much, you were essentially playing a zero-sum game, cutting up the same pie over and over again. You weren't creating anything new. And all the while there were those customers — just waiting to chomp away if you could give them just a nudge to do so.

But did Americans really want to eat more tacos? "We had always viewed ourselves as a kind of 'one-off' brand," Martin recalled in a recent interview. Tacos — or, for that matter, pizza — would always be the second choice to buying a burger. "That caused us to view ourselves as in a small pond — that the competition was other Mexican outlets."

Then Martin met a young marketing genius named Elliot Bloom. A student of the so-called "smart research" trend in Europe, which emphasized the placing of relative "weights" on consumer responses so as to understand what really mattered to a customer, Bloom had completely different ideas about the market for Mexican food. Almost immediately he began running studies on Taco Bell customers. What he found startled: Fast-food consumers were much more sophisticated and open to innovation than previously thought. In fact, they were bored with burgers. Martin loved the idea of competing with McDonald's, and immediately launched a $200 million national ad campaign, the centerpiece of which was a commercial depicting a man threatening to jump off a ledge if he had to eat another hamburger. The results of the campaign were mixed. Sales of some new products, most notably the taco salad, blossomed, but overall customer counts remained vexingly low.

Meantime, Bloom was still playing with consumer surveys, which now revealed something even more surprising: While almost 90 percent of fast-food buyers had already tried Taco Bell, the repeat visit rate of the average consumer was flat. "Reach" wasn't the problem. Frequency was. And when you started studying the customers who *were* coming back — the "heavy users" — price and value — not taste and presentation — were the key. "That was shocking," Martin recalls. "Value was the number-one issue for these guys — and there were a lot of them — 30 percent of our customers accounted for 70 percent of sales. For a lot of us, that was disturbing. Our whole culture was sort of 'out of the kitchen,' you know, the notion that taste, cleanliness, and presentation was the key. But that's not what this new kind of customer was about. His message was loud and clear: more for less. So the business question became — how do you create *more* of these guys?"

One way, of course, was to give them what they wanted. But that was discounting, Martin's financial people warned. "I argued with them. I said, 'Look, this isn't stupid discounting, this is a way to right-price the business after a decade of inflation.'"

Bloom suggested an unscientific test of the idea. Let's not make a lot of national noise about this, he said. Let's go someplace where we might get some clean data. There was, in fact, an ideal place to do so. It was Texas, which in the mid-1980s was suffering from one of the worst recessions the oil patch had seen for decades. "We went in and really cut prices and got a dramatic increase in business," Martin says. "We did not make money but it showed us the potential for upping the number of visits per store."

After Martin widened the test, Bloom reported something even better. "Everyone had thought that if we cut 25 percent off the average price of, say, a taco, that the average check size would drop," Martin says. "I never believed that — that satiety was satiety — and, in fact, I was right. Within seven days of initiating the test, the average check was right back to where it was before — it was just four instead of three items." In other words, the mere presence of more for less induced people to eat more.

To get the profit margins back up, Martin turned to what he knew best: cost-cutting. He fired whole swaths of middle managers, then looked at the stores themselves. In them he found what he called a "just plain weird thing, when you thought about it: 30 percent of the typical Taco Bell store was dining area, 70 percent was kitchen. What was that about?" Martin reversed the ratio, ripping out old-fashioned kitchens and sending the bulk of the cooking to off-site preparation centers.

With his margins back up enough to quell upper management fears, Martin took the value meal concept nationwide in 1988. The response was rapid, dramatic, and, ultimately for Taco Bell, transformative. Between 1988 and 1996 sales grew from $1.6 billion to $3.4 billion.

And the value meal was spreading — to Burger King, to Wendy's, to Pizza Hut and Domino's and just about every player worth its salt except . . . David Wallerstein's McDonald's Corporation.

Not that McDonald's was hurting. Its aggressive advertising and marketing had by the late 1980s turned it into a global force unparalleled in the history of the restaurant business. It could, in a sense, afford to call its own tune. (Or at least deal with PR disasters, as was the case in the late 1980s, when the firm was under attack by nutritionists and public health advocates for its use of saturated fats.) But by 1990, Martin's Taco Bell value meals were taking their toll on McDonald's sales. Worse, McDonald's lack of a value meal had become a hot topic on Wall Street, where its stock was slumping. Analysts were restless. On December 17, 1990, one of them, a sharp-eyed fast-food specialist at Shearson Lehman named Carolyn Levy, gave an uncharacteristically frank interview to a reporter at *Nation's Restaurant News*. "McDonald's must bite the bullet," she said. "Some people I know in Texas told me it's cheaper to take their kids for a burger and fries at Chili's than to take them to McDonald's." In McDonald's board meetings, Wallerstein and his supporters used the bad press to good effect. Two weeks later the front page of the same newspaper read: "MCDONALD'S KICKS OFF VALUE MENU BLITZ!"

Though it is difficult to gauge the exact impact of supersizing upon the appetite of the average consumer, there are clues about it in the now growing field of satiety — the science of understanding human satisfaction. A 2001 study by nutritional researchers at Penn State University, for example, sought to find out whether the presence of larger portions *in themselves* induced people to eat more. Men and women volunteers, all reporting the same level of hunger, were served lunch on four separate occasions. In each session, the size of the main entree was increased, from 500 to 625 to 750 and finally to 1000 grams. After four weeks, the pattern became clear: As portions increased, all participants ate increasingly larger amounts, despite their stable hunger levels. As the scholars wrote: "Subjects consumed approximately 30 percent more energy when served the largest as opposed to the smallest portion." They had documented exactly what John Martin had realized fifteen years earlier: that satiety is not satiety. Human hunger could be expanded by merely offering more and bigger options.

Certainly the best nutritional data suggest so as well. Between 1970 and 1994, the USDA reports, the amount of food available in the American food supply increased 15 percent — from 3300 to 3800 calories or by about 500 calories per person per day. During about the same period (1977–1995), average individual caloric intake increased by almost 200 calories, from 1876 calories a day to 2043 calories a day. One could argue which came first, the appetite or the bigger burger, but the calories — they were on the plate and in our mouths.

By the end of the century, supersizing — the ultimate expression of the value meal revolution — reigned. As of 1996 some 25 percent of the $97 billion spent on fast food came from items promoted on the basis of either larger size or extra portions. A serving of McDonald's french fries had ballooned from 200 calories (1960) to 320 calories (late 1970s) to 450 calories (mid-1990s) to 540 calories (late 1990s) to the present 610 calories. In fact, everything on the menu had exploded in size. What was once a 590-calorie McDonald's meal was now . . . 1550 calories. By 1999 heavy users — people who eat fast food more than twenty times a month and Martin's holy grail — accounted for $66 billion of the $110 billion spent on fast food. Twenty times a month is now McDonald's marketing goal for every fast-food eater. The average Joe or Jane thought nothing of buying Little Caesar's pizza "by the foot," of supersizing that lunchtime burger or supersupersizing an afternoon snack. Kids had come to see bigger everything — bigger sodas, bigger snacks, bigger candy, and even bigger doughnuts — as the norm; there was no such thing as a fixed, immutable size for anything, because anything could be made a lot bigger for just a tad more.

There was more to all of this than just eating more. Bigness: The concept seemed to fuel the marketing of just about everything, from cars (SUVs) to homes (mini-manses) to clothes (super-baggy) and then back again to food (as in the Del Taco Macho Meal, which weighed four pounds). The social scientists and the marketing gurus were going crazy trying to keep up with the trend. "Bigness is addictive because it is about power," commented Irma Zall, a teen marketing consultant, in a page-one story in *USA Today*. While few teenage boys can actually finish a 64-ounce Double Gulp, she added, "it's empowering to hold one in your hand."

The pioneers of supersize had achieved David Wallerstein's dream. They had banished the shame of gluttony and opened the maw of the American eater wider than even they had ever imagined.

3

···················

WORLD WITHOUT
BOUNDARIES

(*Who Let the Calories In*)

SOMETIME DURING the late 1980s — no one can pinpoint the exact date — Ron Magruder, the president of the thriving Olive Garden chain of Italian restaurants, received a telephone call from a dissatisfied customer. The call had been patched all the way up to Magruder because it was so . . . different. The caller, named Larry, wasn't complaining about the food or the service or the prices. Instead, Larry was upset that he could no longer fit into any of the chairs in his local Olive Garden.

"I had to wait more than an hour and half to get a table," Larry told Magruder. "But then I found that there wasn't a single booth or chair where I could sit comfortably."

Magruder, a heavyset man easily moved to enthusiasm, was sympathetic to Larry's plaint. And as president, he could do something about it. He had his staff contact the company that manufactured the chairs for the chain and order a thousand large-size chairs. He then had these distributed, three each, to every Olive Garden restaurant in the nation. It was, as Magruder later told the eminent restaurant business journalist Charles Bernstein, a perfect example of his management philosophy: "We're going to go the extra mile for any customer, no matter what the situation."

Tales like these are the warp and woof of contemporary American management culture, limning as they do the ageless high wisdom that the customer is always right. But the essentials of Larry's tale — the easing of painful, if traditional, boundaries like a restaurant chair, and the acceptance of excess — also go to the core of the popular culture that gave birth to the modern American obesity epidemic. Indeed, if fast-food companies of the 1980s seemed to see the American eater as an endlessly expanding vessel for their product, Americans of the same period rejected the entire notion of limits themselves. They seemed to believe that the old wisdom could be inverted: Gain could come without pain. In 1980 even the hidebound U.S. Department of Agriculture began promoting its new diet guidelines as *The Hassle-Free Food Guide.*

Nowhere did this new boundary-free culture of American food consumption thrive better than in the traditional American family, which by the '80s was undergoing rapid change. The catalyst came in two forms: individual freedom (born of the liberation movements of the '60s and '70s) and entrepreneurial adventurism (born of the economic tumult of the late '70s and early '80s). Women, freed from the stereotypical roles and duties of the '50s housewife, now made up a substantial percentage of the workforce. Taking their rightful place alongside their male counterparts in every profession from law to medicine to construction to engineering, they set forth to transform the American corporation and helped fuel a long overdue renaissance in management culture. Men, freed from the traditional notions of being the family's sole breadwinner and disinclined to give any one employer too much loyalty, went in search of professional and personal fulfillment. Garages burst with strange new contraptions called PCs, and Mom soon joined Pop in founding strange and almost magical new businesses. Freedom was good — and profitable.

The familial price of this freedom was told in time — mainly the lack of it when it came to the kids. And when it came to eating together, that time became ever dearer. The mom of a generation previous had had the time to cook a complete meal, insist that everyone show up to eat it, and then wrestle each child's food issues into an acceptable family standard. The new parent had no time for such unpleasantness. After all, what was more important: to enjoy one's limited time with one's children, dining out at McD's, or to use that time to replicate the parent's own less than idealized childhood table? Most parents were pragmatists. It was easier and more practical simply to eat out — or to order in.

The numbers show that that is exactly what the American family did. In 1970 what the USDA calls the "food away from home" portion of the average American's food dollar was 25 percent; by 1985 it had jumped to 35 percent and by 1996 Americans were spending more than 40 percent of every food dollar on meals obtained away from home. The trend was clear and unambiguous. In 1977 the proportion of meals consumed away from home was 16 percent; by 1987 that figure rose to 24 percent; by 1995 to 29 percent. Snacking too moved out of the home and into the streets, with 17 percent of snacks being consumed away from home in 1977, 20 percent in 1987, and 22 percent in 1995.

Calorically speaking, the shift was even less ambiguous. In 1977, Americans got only 18 percent of their calories away from home; in a decade that figure had grown to 27 percent, and in less than another decade (by 1994) to 34 percent. Fat consumption away from the traditional table soared, from 19 percent of total calories in 1977 to 28 percent in 1987 to 38 percent in 1995. Where fast-food places accounted for just 3 percent of total caloric intake in 1977, that share rose to 12 percent two decades later.

And thanks to the revolution in food processing, commodity prices, and fast-food marketing, what was in that food also changed rapidly. Here the Butzian revolution had fused with the triumph of the value meal and new-style sugar and fat technologies. Yummy sizzling meat — it was everywhere! Coca-Cola —

it was almost free! In this regard the single most telling statistic came from the USDA. "We calculate that if food away from home had the same average nutritional densities as food at home . . . Americans would have consumed 197 fewer calories per day." Put another way, that's an extra pound's worth of energy *every twenty days.*

That food on the run was getting more caloric was a reflection of another, less understood phenomenon, that of "nutrient control." Nutrient control means simply that — the degree to which one exercises some control over what goes into one's food. Fast food and convenience food by their very nature preclude such control; to put it the way a French intellectual might, a Big Mac is a caloric fait accompli. So is a Swanson's TV dinner or any boil-in-the-bag fettuccine Alfredo. To be convenient — to be stable and have a long shelf life, or to retain good "mouthfeel" after an hour under the fast-food heat lamp — food had to contain larger and more condensed amounts of fats and sugars. Such was one source of those extra 197 calories.

But Americans of the 1980s kept eating more for another reason as well. Increasingly, as the away-from-home numbers show, they ate in a kind of gastronomic time warp, justifying their larger portions because they were "eating out" or because it was "a treat." But now the treat had become a daily treat. Eating out was just, well, eating. As three of the USDA's more pointed scholars put it: "Where that may have been a reasonable attitude twenty years ago, when eating out was more infrequent, [today] that belief becomes increasingly inappropriate." Americans had ceded "nutrient control" — and self-control.

Of course, ceding control — avoiding hassles and conflicts with one's children — was the whole point, wasn't it?

Such was the overwhelming message of a wide range of 1980s child-care books, most of which centered on the important but ultimately squishy notions of "autonomy" and "empowerment." Both notions derived from a reaction to the conformist society of the previous generation — the same society that had stereotyped and oppressed woman and made man into little more than a "productive unit." Such books inevitably emphasized the overriding importance of a child's personal choices as a way to instill self-confidence and responsibility. Unfortunately, when it came to food, their authors tended to view the child as a kind of infant-sage, his nutritional whims a "natural" guide to how parents should feed him.

One of the more wide-ranging of these books — one that eventually sold more than 3 million copies and made its authors virtual nutritionist stars — was *Fit for Life*. Published in 1985 and written by Harvey and Marilyn Diamond, two holistic nutritionists from California, *Fit* was originally pitched as a dietary guidebook ("You can eat more kinds of food than you ever ate without counting calories!"). But in the ever conflict-avoiding 1980s, *Fit for Life* eventually became a kind of all-purpose advice book for regaining one's "vital principles." On the subject of children and nutrition, its authors were insistent: Food should never become a dinner-table battleground. "Pressure causes tension," the Diamonds wrote. "Where food is concerned, tension is always to be avoided." Here the operative notion — largely unproven — is that a child restrained from overeating will either rebel by secretly gorging when away from the table or, worse, will suffer such a loss of self-esteem that a lifetime of disastrous eating behaviors will ensue.

The authors of 1985's *Are You Hungry? A Completely New Approach to Raising Children Free of Food and Weight Problems* took the sentiment to its next logical step. With the intent of helping children develop their own sense of self-control, New School for Social Research authors Jane R. Hirschmann and Lela Zaphiropoulos put forth three basic guidelines to parents: "First, they [children] should eat when they are physically hungry and only when they are hungry. Second, they themselves should have the responsibility for determining the foods they eat. And finally they should stop eating when they feel full."

Reading deeper, however, there was also another issue: the comfort of the parent. "To questions like 'Why can't I eat my dessert first?' or 'Why can't I eat all my Halloween candy?' you can answer 'No reason at all. You can.' And this answer doesn't lead to ill health or loss of family discipline," the pair promised. In fact "good parenting requires this answer because it leads to 'self-demand' feeding . . . Life can be much easier with self-demand feeding because it allows you to give up unnecessary control and the concomitant struggles over food."

It would be tempting to lay the entire blame for such intellectual indulgence at the feet of the ever demonized politically correct, but there it does not belong, or at least not entirely, for the fact is that, despite our "spare the rod, spoil the child" big talk, Americans have been historically predisposed in exactly the opposite direction, particularly in matters concerning children and food. Part of this derives from the very nature of the American family. As the sociologist Edward Shorter has noted, in contrast to its European counterpart, the American family was "born modern." From early on it was nuclear, seeking as it did to withdraw itself from the meddling of the traditional extended family. At its center was not a child in the European tradition — essentially just one more actor in an extended community — but rather a child as the very reason for being, for feeling and acting independently. As a result, the American child commanded disproportionate "respect" — he wasn't to be hurried too quickly into the pain of adulthood. Rather, he was to be mollified with the tremendous bounty of the new nation. And the nation's greatest bounty was food, glorious food.

That is, *more* food. For well into the postwar years, when true undernutrition among the middle class became a rarity, undernutrition remained the central concern of most parents. This is not to say that Americans have never attempted to deal with fat children; the pages of turn-of-the-century newspapers were filled with advertisements promising to help one's "chunky" offspring "slim down." But the thrust of those efforts — from early-twentieth-century medicaments to twenty-first-century fat camps — were almost always social and aesthetic: Plump Janey was being alienated at school. Fat Joey was being harassed by the slimmer boys. *Nowhere in those efforts was childhood overeating paired solely with health concerns.* Always in the background were the taunts and the teases. The notion that overfeeding might be over-ridingly a health problem and a health problem alone never entered the American psyche.

A counterpoint to the culture of the overfed American could be found in late-nineteenth-century France, which like the United States of the period was undergoing rising rates of urbanization and declining rates of childhood mortality. The French family too was coming to a new understanding of the child. With wet-nursing on the decline, the French mother was increasingly in charge of her own little *enfant cher.* There was thus more natural sentiment toward the occupant of the cradle. This was a new development, for a new reason. Only a hundred years or so previous there would have been a good chance that little Mathilde, away from her mother's breast, would not make it past her first birthday; true maternal attachments could wait until she was five or six. By the late nineteenth century, however, with better medical practices and pasteurized milk widely available, the chances were good that not only would she make it out of the cradle but that she would be a part of Mama's life for the rest of her years. Chère Mathilde became chère chère Mathilde.

One of the first unanticipated products of this new generation of more indulgent French mothers was *l'enfant obèse.* By the 1930s French medical journals were full of case histories of fat children. But unlike their American counterparts, the French fat child was not considered to be so socially vulnerable. Rather, his or her condition was to be dealt with — directly and forthrightly — as a medical issue. Fortunately, there was already a public health network through which to treat the problem. This was known as the puericulture system.

Puericulture had begun as an informal system of health education in the late nineteenth century, principally to teach new mothers how to prevent and treat tuberculosis, then on the rise. By the early twentieth century, puericulture was adapted to teach better mothering techniques to a new generation of mothers. When the first results of parental overindulgence showed up as a two-hundred-pound teenager (as it did), the advocates of puericulture retooled again. Their prescription: Adults had to take control of a child's diet. Period. If they did not, the child would certainly become a sickling.

Soon, French mothers were being taught a new puericulture dogma. The essentials were this: Plump children were not necessarily a point of pride; mealtimes should be as nearly set in stone as possible; snacks, except on rare occasions, were to be forbidden; second helpings were out of the question, save, perhaps, on a holiday; children should eat separately from adults, so as "to avoid arousing his desires" with richer adult fare. And the child was never to be left to his or her own personal choice. Augusta Moll-Weiss, the mother of puericulture and the founder of the influential Paris School for Mothers, put it thusly: "It is unimportant how much freedom is left in this choice; the essential thing is that the quality and quantity of the diet correspond to the exertion of the young human being." Lastly, all meals should be supervised by an adult. "The basic message was surprisingly persistent," writes the cultural historian Peter N. Stearn, the principal American chronicler of puericulture. "Too much food was bad. Children must learn to discipline their appetites and eating habits, sitting for meals regularly, chewing carefully, expecting adult supervision."

For the French, struggle and tension at the table were simply part of the process of setting reasonable boundaries for children.

About this the Diamonds and the Hirschmanns and their many present-day imitators have had nothing to say. Yet this very lack of pragmatic boundary-setting may well be wreaking nutritional havoc on children.

Consider perhaps the central dogma in the child-as-food-sage theology — that a child "knows" when he or she is full. Such is the belief, repeated emphatically to this day, of many of the nation's leading nutritional authorities, both academic and popular. This despite new research showing that children, just like adults, increasingly do not know when they are full. In a recent study by the Penn State nutrition scholar Barbara Rolls, researchers examined the eating habits of two groups of children, one of three-year-olds, another of five-year-olds. Both groups reported equal levels of energy expenditure and hunger. The children were then presented with a series of plates of macaroni and cheese. The first plate was a normal serving built around age-appropriate baseline nutritional needs; the second plate was slightly larger; the third was what we might now call "supersized." The results were both revealing and worrisome. The younger children consistently ate the same baseline amount, leaving more and more food on the plate as the servings grew in size. The five-year-olds acted as if they were from another planet, devouring whatever was put on their plates. Something had happened. As was the case with their adult counterparts in another of Rolls's studies (cited in chapter 2), the mere presence of larger portions had induced increased eating. Far from trusting their own (proverbial and literal) guts, children, the author concluded, should instead get "clear information on appropriate portion sizes."

Theorizing aside, the continuing disinclination to restrain a child's eating flies in the face of overwhelming evidence that, of all age groups, children seem to be the ones who respond best to clear dietary advice. In four randomized studies of obese six- to twelve-year-olds, those offered frequent, simple behavioral advice — in other words those who were lovingly "hassled" — were substantially less overweight ten years later than those who did not get the advice. And thirty of those children were no longer obese at all.

The case for early intervention has been further buttressed by new studies on another age-old medical injunction: Never put a child on a diet. For decades, the concern was that such undernutrition could lead to stunted growth. But the authors of a study of 1062 children under age three have concluded differently. Writing in the journal *Pediatrics,* they state that "a supervised, low-saturated-fat and low-cholesterol diet has no influence on growth during the first three years of life." And overweight children who were put on such a diet ended up with better, more moderate eating habits, to boot.

In other words, it's good to tell Johnny when enough is enough.

Another way to find out where food intake minus mitigation leads is simply to look at the food world that children were "allowed" to create, a world that can be summarized by one word: snacking.

In the 1980s, snacking was flat-out encouraged. The first to do so were the decade's ever more economically busy parents, who simply wanted to make sure that their kids ate *something.* Fair enough. But snacking was also indirectly encouraged by new understandings in nutritional science, which suggested that many people, and particularly children, needed to eat more than three meals a day. Although such insights have a strong basis in fact, their real-world utility was often twisted by the media and food companies. Suddenly it was "unnatural" to eat three times a day. Progressive people ate "when their bodies told them to." Snacking was not only not bad; it was good to eat all day long. Such was the message of the diet craze known as "grazing," a quasi-regimen endlessly fawned over and packaged by the mainstream media.

Food companies, of course, were happy to join in the party. There would be "Snack Good," "Snack Healthy," and, by the early 1990s, "SnackWell." And with sugar and fat prices lower than ever, it was easy for new, less bridled players to share the fun and profit. The number and variety of high-calorie snack foods and sweets soared; where all through the 1960s and 1970s the number of yearly new candy and snack products remained stable — at about 250 a year — that number jumped to about 1000 by the mid-1980s and to about 2000 by the late 1980s. The rate of new, high-calorie bakery foods also jumped substantially. A revealing graphic of this trend, charted against the rise in obesity rates, was published by the *American Journal of Clinical Nutrition* in 1999; the two lines rise in remarkable tandem.

The increased variety in snacks and sweets enabled by the Butzian revolution in agriculture conjured a new and ever fattening pattern of eating. Just as the presence of supersized portions had stimulated Americans to eat more at mealtime, the *sheer presence* of a large variety of new high-calorie snacks was deeply reshaping the *overall habits* of the American eater. Studying the eating patterns of adults, and using the most advanced monitoring and tracking systems available, researchers at the USDA Human Nutrition Research Center at Tufts University were able to document an amazing phenomenon: The higher the variety of snack foods present in their subjects' diets, the higher the number of calories from those foods they would consume, and the higher would be the subjects' consequent body fatness. This was stunning. Historically, the drive to eat a variety of food had been a positive element in human evolution, helping early humans to increase *and* balance fuel intake, and, consequently, improve their metabolic, physical, and mental abilities. The drive for novelty had been healthful. Now the same drive had become unhealthful. "Today," the Tufts researchers noted, "a drive to overeat when variety is plentiful is disadvantageous for weight regulation because dietary variety is greater than ever before and comes primarily from energy-dense commercial foods rather than from the energy-poor but micronutrient-rich vegetables and fruit for which the variety principle originally evolved." In short, variety had become the enemy.

You could see the phenomenon everywhere you went. One of the more insidious of the new snacks appeared in California, where the Snak Club company began selling huge (as much as five portions) but inexpensive ($.99) bags of unbranded candy. The bags were routinely placed near checkout stands, where a telling ad campaign forthrightly proclaimed that the bag of candy just within Junior's reach was "a meal in itself." Ten years later the label was changed to "a treat in itself."

And snack kids did. In the '80s, in every single age group, between-meal chomping was louder than ever. Moreover, the troubling tendency to snack several times every day — in essence making snacking part of a de facto meal pattern — was perpetuating itself into adolescence and young adulthood. To find out how much so, the pre-eminent nutrition scholar Barry Popkin and his associates at the University of North Carolina at Chapel Hill studied the dietary patterns of 8493 nineteen- to twenty-nine-year-olds over the period 1977–1996. The results showed that not only had snacking prevalence soared, but so had the number of snacks per day and the number of calories per snacking occasion.

The demographics of increased snacking also revealed a new and disturbing trend: The most avid snackers were the poor. In the same period the snacking rate per day among low-income households went from 67 percent to 82 percent. Snacking by whites increased the least while snacking by Hispanics and African Americans increased the most. The greatest increases were in the poor-to-middle-class South. And like meals in fast-food joints, the caloric density of snacks was growing. As Popkin concluded, "This large increase in total energy and energy density of snacks among young adults in the U.S. may be contributing to our obesity epidemic."

Beyond the immediate contribution of more calories to the diet, the very nature of modern snacking may be pushing children toward obesity. New studies show that, far from the romanticized "eat when you feel like it" philosophy, eating more often in itself may make one fat, regardless of the calorie count. In a recent summary paper in the British medical journal *Lancet,* the scholars Gary Frost and Anne Dornhorst explained: "Not only did hunter-gatherers eat a diet low in fat and derived mainly from slowly absorbed carbohydrates, but also by eating less frequently they spent long periods of the day post-absorptively [fasting.] Today's grazing culture results in a disproportionate amount of time being spent post-prandially, which favors glycogen synthesis and fat disposition."

In other words, a perpetually snacking child — whether he knows best or not — is literally a walking, talking, fat-making machine. One that knows no limits.

If the parents of the early '80s had, in essence, let the calories in, they would soon be aided in doing so by a most unlikely accomplice: the public school system.

Until the mid-'70s, public high schools were still a bastion of traditional postwar culture, a place where the boundaries, however frayed, still held. In postwar America, a teacher's ability to act under the legal cover of *in loco parentis* was rarely questioned. Hence, at least on campus, teachers wielded broad cultural influence. This was because a teacher was, for the most part, assumed to be acting in the best interests of the child. The arch of his eyebrow or the pursing of her lip meant something. School was their empire.

A second standard-bearer of campus life concerned food. Nutritionally, the cafeteria of the '70s still reigned as the center of activity for those cool enough to have parents who didn't — or couldn't, or wouldn't — pack a lunch for them. There were Coke machines, but they were few and they dispensed a mere six to eight ounces at a time, and were peripheral to campus life, the places where amateur smokers cadged a quick one between classes.

Such, at least, were the lingering images of public schools held by many '80s parents, who were (sometimes consciously and often not) hoping that the duties they no longer had time for at home might somehow be fulfilled at school.

By the time Me Generation parents began handing their children over to the schools, though, the empire had changed. The broad, boundary-imposing authority of the teacher crumbled under cultural, legal, and economic attack. The old, wide-ranging interpretation of *in loco parentis* had been eroded by court case after court case. Many of these turned around the issue of free speech — something Me Generation parents held particularly dear. (And perhaps even dearer since many of the high school speech cases involved the "symbolic free speech value" of wearing one's hair long.) Other legal findings limited the ability of teachers to discipline students — corporally or otherwise. The net effect of such schoolroom jurisprudence — and of the constant hectoring and second-guessing from society in general — was to make the teacher hunker down and back off. As Thomas R. McDaniel wrote in his 1983 essay "The Teacher's Ten Commandments," the best thing a truly concerned teacher could do was simple: "Sign up for a course in school law."

The final blow to the old empire came in the form of budgetary cutbacks. Ironically, many of these were supported by — if not originated by — the very same generation that was now hoping for the old system to come through just one more time. Their support for California's Proposition 13 was a case in point.

Fueled by inflation and rising property taxes, the 1979 ballot measure required a 1 percent cap on all property tax increases. Its principal proponent, a cigar-chomping Orange County businessman named Howard Jarvis, was a longtime anti-tax activist with a penchant for public speaking. As a small businessman and property owner himself, Jarvis easily connected to the growing legions of "Invisible Americans" — the same folk, many of them traditional Democrats, who had grown tired of government inefficiency and overtaxation and who would, only a year later, elect Ronald Reagan president. Persuasively Jarvis argued their case: If property taxes weren't capped, the very people who had helped build the Golden State would no longer be able to live in their own modest postwar tract homes. The measure's opponents — they were, in truth, few — took a different tack. Proposition 13, they claimed, would bring an end to the Golden State itself; it would destroy quality education, not to mention the vast network of public services that so many Californians had come to take for granted.

In all of this ran a variant of the generational temper tantrum that Earl Butz had encountered only a few years earlier. The folk wanted what they wanted when they wanted it. Proposition 13 passed in a 2–1 landslide. As did its imitators in twenty other states.

Although budget surpluses initially softened many of the budget cuts feared by the measures' opponents, Proposition 13 and its copycats did lead to many important cuts in the schools. Physical education, for one, was gutted (see chapter 4). There were closings and reduced hours at the many public libraries upon which so many schools depended. Perhaps most important, education was no longer considered the great untouchable in discussions of public spending.

In California, where famously well-funded schools had long enjoyed *primus inter pares* status, school cafeterias felt the first pinch, and the way they reacted to it foreshadowed how school lunch programs nationwide would deal with similar cuts.

In 1981 the California Department of Education ended its successful Food Service Equipment Program. For decades the program had augmented local school budgets by providing millions of dollars for the maintenance and upgrading of school cafeterias. For the Los Angeles Unified School District (LAUSD), then experiencing unprecedented growth, the cut "was a huge blow," says Laura Chinnock, now the assistant director of the district's mammoth food services department. "What that did was to force us to make changes in the existing infrastructure instead of expanding. So now we had to feed, say, two thousand kids through the old service windows that were built to service half that. Well, now double *that* — and keep in mind that the minimum legal amount of time for a child to eat lunch is twenty minutes — and you'll see why now some big schools have kids lining up at ten-thirty in the morning for lunch."

Try as they might, the period's food service directors could not make a cafeteria that once cooked for five hundred cook for five thousand. As Gene White, one of the state's most respected school nutritionists and a longtime policy hand, says, "If the school cafeteria couldn't cook the meals, the natural alternative was to get rid of a lot of the traditional cafeteria's functions. In the '80s, that meant what you might call outsourcing — cooking the meals someplace else and bringing them in to be reheated, or actually contracting with an outside source to deliver pre-plated meals." However one looked at it, the public school had lost control of many of the ingredients that went into that food. "Those pre-plated meals must meet some standard, but the overall quality is much like a TV dinner," says White. "I'll leave you to decide what that means."

Yet even outsourcing would fail to cure the cafeteria's chronic blues. Food service budgets simply failed to keep pace with growing school populations. Part of the problem was political. Not only did schools now have to compete for money with all other public services — the legacy of Jarvis — they increasingly had to do so without what was once their most politically influential supporter: middle-class parents, who were now defecting in droves to private schools. There was a cultural problem as well. With fast-food joints proliferating faster than ever, students were more and more likely to bypass the cafeteria completely and, when no one was looking, simply bolt from campus to McD's, rules to the contrary or no. Food service departments around the nation bled. Slowly but surely many came to the inevitable conclusion: Food service departments would have to become more entrepreneurial.

Fast-food makers had also come to a similar conclusion, for different reasons, but with very similar ends. For a decade firms like Taco Bell and Pizza Hut had tried — with occasional success — to develop institutional feeding programs. One way to do that was to sell frozen versions of their most popular products to large institutions. But frozen entrees never quite captured the imagination, let alone the taste buds, of increasingly sophisticated pizza chompers. Worst, to make the effort really work, fast-food makers would have to spend a great deal of money reformulating their products to meet USDA limits on fats and sugars in school lunch foods. And that conjured even more corporate dyspepsia: What would happen to their overall brand image if those reformulated products didn't taste as good as those plied by the same company's franchisees just down the street? Would that drive down regular sales as well? There had to be a way — but where was it?

The answer came in the early 1990s, when a group of enterprising Pizza Hut salespeople asked: Why not — instead of trying to qualify Pizza Hut pizzas under the school lunch program — find a way to sell the pizzas outside of the federally regulated cafeterias, say, out on the lawn, or on the playground, or even over by the old vending machine areas? The executives took the idea to several large school districts. One of them was Los Angeles Unified. There, as one nutrition director says, "it was as if this huge light bulb went on." Not only could the district get out of the never ending battles with the USDA and Pizza Hut over reformulation, it could also make some money on its own by purchasing the pizzas centrally and then selling them at a markup. And by offering a branded product, they might additionally keep students off the streets and on campus.

As it would evolve, the deal came with a number of other perks as well. Fast-food companies helped underwrite the purchase of zippy new "food carts," to be placed strategically about the campus during lunch and break time — in essence becoming the new food service equipment program. There were added incentives for schools that sold the pizzas at glee club meetings and for those who used them for campus fund-raisers.

But the single most important innovation was the way in which individual schools actually got the pizzas. It worked like this: Every morning the school's cafeteria manager would estimate how many pizzas — or tacos, or burritos — the "non-cafeteria eaters" would likely consume that day. The manager would then call a designated local Pizza Hut franchisee and place the order. Just before lunch the franchisee would deliver the piping-hot pies to cafeteria workers, who would load them into the shining Pizza Hut food carts and send them off to the waiting students. In the parlance of management, it was a win-win situation: Schools had found a way to feed kids economically and to keep them on campus; fast-food companies got a toehold in a market that had been unreachable — and without the expense of having to obey the law. The students? They got an opportunity to eat . . . the same food that more and more of them were eating at home. By 1999, 95 percent of 345 California high schools surveyed by the nonprofit Public Health Institute were offering branded fast foods as *à la carte* entree items for lunch. At 71 percent of those schools, fast food made up a substantial portion of total food sales — up to 70 percent. Seventy-two percent of the same schools permitted fast-food and beverage advertising on campus.

But what really was wrought? Who really was served? Certainly anti–fast-food activists now had a genuine beef with school administration. Not only had "the system" found a way around the well-intended (and very healthy) USDA guidelines, it had also instigated another problem: dietary overconsumption. Portion sizes for pizza were a case in point. The cafeteria dispensed individual pizzas that, by law, corresponded to USDA portion recommendations. In the LAUSD, for example, a typical individual school lunch pizza runs somewhere around 5.5 ounces. A typical food cart, or branded, pizza — sold outside the cafeteria and thus unrestrained by such regulation — weighs in at almost twice that. The school lunch pizza had 375 calories, the branded "personal" pizza more than twice that — almost one-third of the recommended daily calories for a typical American teenager. The schools had lost control of calories.

Among obesity-minded nutritionists, such was clearly cause for concern. But now the school district was hooked. Concerned about the enormous calorie count, Laura Chinnock, the LAUSD veteran, went back to Pizza Hut reps and proposed that the food cart pizza be just slightly reformulated — "just use some lower-fat cheese, for example." She was immediately rebuffed. "The concern was that somehow that would affect the taste — and that would somehow taint the overall Pizza Hut product. Kids might not buy so much of it on the way home or for dinner, say." Chinnock repeatedly took the issue up with her superiors at LAUSD, but with the nation's largest and most tumultuous school system in a constant budgetary crisis, anything that might cost money simply did not make it onto the agenda.

But something else had happened as well — something no one, save, likely, the Pizza Hut people, had seen: The food carts — the latter-day successors to the dingy old vending areas — had become "cool." Whatever they purveyed had cachet — it sold and sold and sold and sold. Intrigued by this, Chinnock one day decided to try an experiment. Without telling students, teachers, or Pizza Hut vendors, she substituted USDA-formulated pizzas for the usual branded pizzas. "The response was nil — they gobbled them up just like usual," she recalls. "They were basically eating the brand."

By the mid-1990s school principals had also joined the brand-fest. Faced with continuing shortfalls in funds for sports teams, academic clubs, plant upkeep, and even janitorial services, they were a receptive audience to new overtures from the soft drink industry. This time the inducements came in the form of "pouring contracts." Such contracts typically involved three monetary perks for three contractual promises. For agreeing to sell only, say, Coke, a school would receive commissions and a yearly bonus payment — sometimes as much as $100,000 — to do with as it liked. In return for putting up Coke advertising around the campus, the school would receive free product to sell at fund-raising events. And in return for making the company's carbonated beverages available during all hours, Coke would provide additional "marketing" tools — banners, posters, etc. — to aid still more school fund-raising events. In a time of tight funds and rising expectations, such contracts proved enormously popular. In Los Angeles, sports-minded parents became some of the biggest advocates of pouring contracts. It is doubtful, however, that those same parents had any clue about what soft drinks were doing to their children's overall diets, not to mention health.

Between 1989 and 1994 consumption of soft drinks by kids soared. The USDA estimated that the proportion of adolescent boys and girls consuming soft drinks on any given day increased by 74 percent and 65 percent, respectively. In many ways the pattern reflected the adult population, where, between 1989 and 1994, soda consumption jumped from 34.7 to 40.3 gallons a year. But the kids were doing something with the soda that few people initially understood: They were drinking it in place of milk and other important nutrient-rich foods.

Worse, they were not compensating for those extra empty calories when they sat down for regular meals. A joint study by Harvard University and Boston Children's Hospital researchers in February 2001 concluded that such excess liquid calories inhibited the ability of older children to compensate at mealtime, leading to caloric imbalance and, in time, obesity. "Compensation for energy consumed in liquid form, which can be observed in very young children (4–5 years)," reviewers of the study concluded, "is lost rapidly in the following years."

When it came to food — and particularly when it came to setting boundaries on its consumption — family and school were hardly alone as they drifted through the 1980s. That other great arbiter of modern life, the media, was also at sea.

For most of the postwar period, the publishers of American diet books were a somewhat predictable lot. While editors might occasionally publish a celebrity diet or a quirky new fitness regimen, the general approach of diet books to weight loss mirrored what physicians, scientists, and nutritionists had always advised: to maintain weight one had to balance calories in with calories out. To lose it, one had to consume fewer and expend more. The lone dissenter was a Cornell University–trained physician named Robert C. Atkins. In 1972 Atkins published a small book that turned conventional wisdom on its head. Instead of counting calories, and always thinking about what one couldn't have, a person who really wanted to lose weight had to find a way to do so pleasantly. And Atkins had found the way.

The way, in fact, was simple — and, as Atkins never failed to note, very scientific. Human beings, he would begin, need three basic nutrients — proteins, fats, and carbohydrates. Once inside the body, proteins were broken down to replenish muscles and tissues, fats were burned or stored for future energy use, and carbohydrates were burned for immediate energy needs. The carbohydrates that didn't get used — and this was key to the Atkins diet — were stored by the liver as glycogen, which was then stored as fat. If the body did not get enough carbohydrates during the day, it would eventually begin to "burn" its fat stores. It was that last bit of information that could make all the difference for the frustrated dieter, Atkins said. If one deprived the body of carbohydrates — sugars — one could "trick" the body into burning its own fat stores. The added bonus of such a system was that one could consume all the fats and proteins one wanted, since the revved-up Atkinized body would either use them for muscle or burn them away.

Not surprisingly, the book, *Dr. Atkins' Diet Revolution,* went to the top of the charts.

Yet much of mainstream publishing remained wary of Atkins. Some old-time editors and critics knew that such a diet had been proffered, on and off, ever since the mid-nineteenth century, when it was popularized by a retired London undertaker named William Banting. Banting, who lost some fifty pounds on the regimen, had published a pamphlet, *On Corpulence,* that had eventually caught the eye of late-nineteenth-century Americans. In the intervening century, the Banting "scheme," as it was inevitably called, had popped up with astounding regularity about every twenty-five years. At one point it was even listed as a "cure" for obesity in the *Merck Manual,* the prestigious physician's handbook.

The nutritionally savvy knew something else about the Banting-Atkins scheme: It was full of medical mumbo jumbo and fraught with potential peril for anyone who followed it for a sustained period of time. It was true that the body stored excess carbohydrates as fat, for example, but it was not so clear that depriving the body of carbohydrates induced the revved-up, fat-burning state that Atkins claimed. It was also unclear what medical consequences flowed from consuming enormous amounts of fat and protein. Gout — something long considered erased in modern times — was an ongoing concern.

But perhaps the biggest objection to the diet was that in the early 1970s the great mass of people simply could not afford to substitute meat for the bulkier — and stomach-filling — meal components like bread and potatoes.

As the 1980s dawned in the major New York houses, two forces colluded to erase the old editors' reluctance to promote "all the meat you want." For one, meat prices were now increasingly within the reach of the average Joe. Butz's revolution in commodity prices had seen to that. Eating a giant hamburger patty and cheese three times a day, or "all the bacon and pork rinds you can," was actually economically viable.

The other factor was publishing itself. The older, medically attuned editors were either retiring or, worse, facing increased pressure to come up with hot new diet books. If they didn't, they were told, someone else would. Calories in, calories out — that was not only boring, but the franchise for it had also been virtually sewed up by Weight Watchers. It was time to offer a bold new category of diet books — or risk losing the opportunity to the newly competitive alternative diet publishers like Atkins and his imitators.

The result was not only an outpouring of Atkins-like low-carb diets, but a like-style gusher of other "all you can eat" diets.

In 1989 W. W. Norton published *The T-Factor Diet*, inverting Atkins's claim and instead focusing on fat as the villain. The book promised that one could "Lose Weight Safely and Quickly Without Cutting Calories — or Even Counting Them!" The key, author Martin Katahn wrote, was something called the "thermogenic effect," the ability of certain foods, in this case not protein as in Atkins but instead carbohydrates, to "rev up" one's fat-burning engine. Although the idea of a thermogenic effect had been hotly debated by scientists and diet pill makers for decades, Katahn and his editors decided to render it as fact. "It is primarily fat in your diet that determines your body fat, and protein and carbohydrate calories don't really matter very much," Katahn wrote. "Once you start replacing some of that fat with carbohydrates you will unlock your body's hidden fat-burning potential: that's the T-factor at work!"

In 1993 Dean Ornish, a California heart specialist who had reported remarkable results reversing heart disease by having patients follow a very low fat diet, joined the all-you-can-eat bandwagon. Now, instead of prescribing his extremely low fat diet for medical patients, he enlarged its prescriptions to a larger audience. As his book jacket described it: "Dr. Ornish's program takes a new approach, one scientifically based on the type of food rather than the amount of food. Abundance rather than hunger and deprivation — so you can eat more frequently, eat a greater quantity of food, and still lose weight and keep it off!"

By 1995, however, Atkinism was back again, this time retooled by HarperCollins and Barry Sears. Reacting to the growing obesity statistics despite the early 1990s consensus that it was fat and not carbs that was the villain, Sears went back to a low-carb basic: "Basta with pasta!" he proclaimed. And forget about exercising too. If one only mixed the right foods, why, "you can burn more fat watching TV than by exercising," he idiotically promised. That same year Bantam introduced Michael and Mary Dan Eades and their notion of "Protein Power," in which one could "eat all the foods you love — steaks, bacon and burgers, cheese and eggs."

The point, of course, is not that the publishing industry and its new ancillary industries in the diet supplement and video sectors were publishing pure schlock (although most of it was). There had been legitimate scientific debate about such things as thermogenesis, fat metabolism, and the metabolic effects of various foods since the mid-nineteenth century, when French scientists like Claude Bernard first discovered the glycogenic (glucose-making) function of the human liver. The point is what the new diets did *not* say. For completely missing from the new genre was one increasingly strange and distant concept: self-control.

The very notion of self-control was anathema to the new generation of diet books. A diet — even a weight loss diet — was no longer about limits to one's gratification. Instead, the subtext was one of scientific entitlement. After all, if one had worked so hard to get so far in one's career, well, how could self-control *really* be an issue? To even suggest such was to make fat a moral issue — and how appropriate was that? No, it was all a matter of using nutritional science to "trick" the body into doing what it should be doing anyway.

The new boundary-free notions about consumption weren't purely the provenance of diet books. In the South and in the Midwest, where conservative Christians had long valued such notions as self-control and personal responsibility, something was amiss as well — namely, a certain sin known as gluttony, which had somehow gotten a good name.

To be fair, it had never had a very bad one — at least not in the United States and not in most Protestant denominations. The seven deadly sins — those were largely Catholic notions, wrapped up as they were with papist ideas of sin and church-administered sacraments. (It says something that one of the most foreign-seeming things in the recent hit movie *Chocolat* was the obsession of the little French town's pious Catholic elder with the sin of gluttony.)

Yet the sin of overconsumption *was* something that had preoccupied a number of American clerics over the years. The early nineteenth century's Sylvester Graham, a Presbyterian minister and the inventor of the graham cracker, had regularly attacked overeating as the source of moral turpitude. As Graham saw it, overeating was a form of overstimulation, which could lead to no end of sinful behaviors.

Later anti-gluttons took a more pragmatic tack. In the 1950s, Charles Shedd, another Presbyterian, wrote a book entitled *Pray Your Weight Away*. Its message was simple: God did not make man to be fat. "When God first dreamed you into creation," Shedd wrote, "there weren't one hundred pounds of excess avoirdupois hanging around your belt." By being fat one was cutting oneself off from the joy that Christ had died to confer on us all. Shedd thus proposed a series of prayer-based activities designed to right the imbalance. There were mealtime affirmations like "Today my body belongs to God. Today I live for him. Today I eat with him." There was faith-based physical exercise. One involved fifteen minutes of karate kicks, executed while reciting the third chapter of Proverbs; another required one to time one's sits-ups to the spoken rhythm of Psalm 19. As R. Marie Griffith, the author of *God's Daughters: Evangelical Women and the Power of Submission,* observes, Shedd was particularly noteworthy because "he balanced his moral rebuke with positive thinking." His message persisted well into the early 1970s, when he published *The Fat Is in Your Head.*

By then things in the American congregation were changing. Fundamentalism brought with it a revival of biblical literalism, and the view that the spiritual world is split between the soul and the body. This worldview had a strange effect on the priority one placed on such things as fatness or thinness, let alone general health. As the Christian journal *Communique* noted in 2000, "Literalists are prone to view biblical texts denouncing 'the flesh' as references to the human body, instead of as symbolic of our human sin nature. Thus, they reason that since the body is evil and mortal, and the soul good and immortal, our priority is to nurture the soul, even if it means neglecting the body." With their reliance placed firmly on a personal Savior, the new conservative Christians also tended to be more fatalistic when it came to illness; He would take care of them, fat or thin. And fat — that seemed to come more naturally.

It was also politically pragmatic. For the leaders of many American congregations, the challenge of the era was competing with the permissiveness rising in secular America. That meant "a little bit o' sugar," as one pastor recalls. Along with literalist, moral preaching about things like homosexuality and abortion would come a new tolerance for "the little sins." (Later on, when many of the new leaders had had their own personal failings televised widely, this doctrine became self-protective as well.) New seminarians were thus told that "holding the flock together" meant accentuating similarities. The same thing was taking place within more liberal circles. At places like Fuller Seminary in Pasadena, California, the student bookstore carried more titles about self-acceptance than it did about traditional moral failings. (Asked where a book about gluttony or sloth might be shelved, a visitor was told: "Where else? In self-help.") The end result of this reorientation, as Marie Griffith says, was that "the American church became like therapy. It was suddenly all about love and tolerance and acceptance, not about individual discipline."

There is, of course, a societal cost to religion's abandonment of the little sins. Religion, like belts or modest meal portions or argumentative family dinners, is a maker of boundaries. Religious beliefs generate the development of moral communities, which, in turn, serve to guide and constrain the action of individuals. As the sociologist Émile Durkheim observed early in the twentieth century, without a religion's "system of interdicts," a society will flounder. (Toynbee agreed, albeit in a secular manner, by noting that the disintegration of a civilization is always marked by "a surrender to a sense of promiscuity.") The relevant point here is clear. If, as Durkheim concluded, God and society "are only one," can there ever be a little sin, at least where religion is concerned?

By the '90s, with such purely theological considerations aside, scholars who studied the sociology of religion began to notice a growing trend: Not only did religion no longer address overconsumption, it seemed somehow implicated in just the opposite — in aiding and abetting overeating. In a 1998 study looking at 3500 U.S. adults, the Purdue University sociologist Kenneth F. Ferraro sought to find out the answer to two interrelated questions: One, was religion related to body weight, especially obesity, and two, did religion intensify, mitigate, or counterbalance the effects of body weight on well-being? To the first, the answer was qualified: Obesity was highest in states where religious affiliation was highest, but the specific differences in body weight between groups were more likely explained by differences in class, ethnicity, and marital status. Of all the religious groups surveyed, Southern Baptists were heaviest, followed by Fundamentalist and Pietistic Protestants. Catholics fell at the middle of the list, while the lowest average body weight was found among Jews and non-Christians. Surveying attitudes within those groups, Ferraro concluded that obesity was associated with higher levels of religiosity. If one calculated in the fact that many of these believers were also of low socioeconomic status, one could almost conclude that eating and religion had become a unified coping strategy. "Consolation and comfort from religion and from eating," Ferraro wrote, "may be a couple of the few pleasures accessible to populations which are economically and politically deprived."

To the second question — did modern religion act to *inhibit* gluttony or obesity — the answer was more surprising. It didn't. Instead, the church had become a nest of unqualified social acceptance. As Ferraro wrote: "There is no evidence of religion operating as a moral constraint on obesity." Instead, Ferraro went on, "higher religious practice was more common among overweight persons, perhaps reflecting religion's emphasis upon tolerating human weakness and its emphasis upon other forms of deviancy such as alcoholism, smoking and sexual promiscuity."

Ferraro warned that it wasn't that religion indirectly promoted higher body weight. Rather, most pastors simply saw obesity and overeating as too risky a subject. "They feel they would risk alienating the flock — at least at this point," says Ferraro. "In that sense we are in a stage with obesity like we were with smoking in the 1950s and 1960s."

And so when it came to overeating, gluttony, and obesity, Christians, like everyone else in America, were in deep, deep denial. As Jerry Falwell said when he heard about Ferraro's findings, "I know gluttony is a bad thing. But I don't know many gluttons."

Family, school, culture, religion — in the late twentieth century, the figurative belt had not only been loosened, it had come off. But what of the literal belt? What of the most traditional measure — and reminder — of excess girth?

While it was true that Americans had been dressing more casually for much of the '60s and '70s, it was also true that they had retained a notion that a good public figure was a lean public figure. High and, more important, middle fashion certainly promoted that, particularly the ultra-slim fashions of the disco years. Jeans companies, particularly Levi Strauss, had not only serviced those inclinations but also helped to create them. The firm's ultra-slim cuts of the late 1970s were so ubiquitous as to inspire caricature in a number of teen movies. A typical scene took place in a Valley jeans boutique, where the jeans were so slim — and the girls so determined to wear them — that they all had to lie down on the floor and wiggle like worms in order to get into the tiny pants.

By the mid-1980s, however, both Levi Strauss and its new competitor, the Gap, had retooled their sizing. Market research had shown that the boomers — the spenders — were getting larger, and, typically, that they did not want to be reminded of their largeness. Nearly overnight, the ultra-slim cuts were gone. In fact, what was once a *regular* cut was now a "slim cut." And now came a whole slew of "new" cuts. A person who wore, say, a size 34 waist and 32 length in a traditional jean could now pick from at least four options: regular fit, easy fit, loose fit, and baggy fit. The unspoken reality of all these new cuts — something everyone knew and everyone winked at — was this: The new cuts were in reality simply bigger sizes, without the bigger numbers.

By the '90s this trend was joined by a number of upstart purveyors of so-called street fashion. Taking their cue from the baggy pants–prison garb of the nation's rap stars — many of them not just fat but morbidly obese — such enterprises prided themselves on making "fat" into "phat." Phat, they would proclaim, was really about empowerment — about rejecting mainstream notions about power and fashion and conformity. "We about a buncha obese playboys!" proclaimed the rap star Big Pun in 1999. It didn't hurt that the same attitude also sold millions of records.

But the same attitude was also a tremendous enabler. Consider Big Pun's story. Pun — his real name was Chris Rios — had by the mid-1990s risen from obscurity in the Bronx to become one of the most promising of a new generation of Latino rap stars. Along the way, his girth had ballooned, from about 220 in the early 1990s to about 400 in the mid-1990s. The man who discovered him, the rap star Fat Joe, saw an advantage to that. "A lot of Latinos and blacks are overweight, so they could relate to this guy," he recalls. "A lot of people think that beautiful is trim and fit, but it ain't. It's what's inside. That's off the rack." The record company that eventually signed Pun, Loud Records, used his round image in their promotions, retooling the slim Michael Jordan figure in the Air Nike ads to one featuring a short round body.

By 1998 Pun had ballooned to 500 pounds. His records were hotter than ever. As typically happens with a young, charismatic star — one thinks, for example, of John Belushi — he was soon surrounded by yes-men and yes-women. The yes-men and the yes-women brought him not drugs but food. "They got him whatever he wanted," one family member recalls. "If we went out to

McDonald's, it would be fifty dollars' worth of food for the whole group, and about twenty of that would be our portion of the bill, and then he would be eating our food as well." A friend recalls how those catering to Pun buttressed his sense of denial about his obesity. "People would tie his shoes for him, or push him around in a wheelchair when he didn't feel like walking, or buy him clothes and hide what size they were," she says. "If he was a size 10xx, people would buy him three to five sizes bigger, so he'd never know how much he was gaining."

And gain Pun did. By the time he was twenty-nine, when he died of a massive heart attack, he weighed 698 pounds. "That was a big shock," says the same family member, "because everyone in rap is always dying from violence and then we're told that he died because of his eating!"

At the suburban mall, the enablers were not rap and baggy pants but rather clothes made with Lycra spandex, a postwar synthetic that the aspirant classes had long considered déclassé to the extreme. No longer. Thanks to the health club boom and the incessant marketing of Olympic stars who wore tight spandex during their televised athletic triumphs, everyone thought they could wear the stuff. Particularly the middle-aged. It felt so . . . good. And didn't it kind of make one look . . . slimmer?

Well, no. At least not if one were from beyond the American mall. Consider the experience of Johannes Hebebrand, a professor of physiology from the University of Marburg in Germany. Hebebrand, whose specialty is obesity and its social origins, was visiting New York in the late 1990s as part of a series of studies he was conducting about social stigma and its psychological effect on the obese. His operative notion was that since fashion magazines and movies had so glorified thinness — and denigrated fatness — that fat people would be less likely to present themselves *as fat* in public. Such was his thesis.

But stepping off the plane and into the nation's shopping malls, Hebebrand was "floored" — what he was seeing was exactly the opposite. "I mean, here were all of these women, wearing this kind of tight black stretch thing!" Hebebrand recalls. "They were huge — their bellies and their derrieres were almost comic-book-sized! I was shocked because in Germany people who are that fat just don't go out. They don't go out because of the shame. But it wasn't the case here in the U.S."

In recent years, big sizes have become an increasingly necessary part of any clothing company's survival strategy. Large sizes account for a growing segment of the total clothing market, rising from about 7.5 percent in 1995 to about 9.4 percent in 2000. Sales of women's sizes 16 and up have risen steadily since 1997, with a 22.2 percent jump between 1999 and 2000. Moreover, the new big sizes are no longer confined to the plus-size sections of major department stores. The Gap, for example, recently nudged up its selections to a size 16, as has the ultra-trendy sportswear label FUBU. Tommy Hilfiger has plans to launch a plus-size line. And in mid-2001, the edgy retailer known as Hot Topic, with 291 stores nationwide, opened its first store for sizes 14 to 26. The firm estimates that about 30 percent of young women in the United States wear a size 14 or bigger. "This is one of the hot new target audiences," says Candace Corlett, a partner with WSL Strategic Retail, a consulting firm in Manhattan. "The population has grown heavier; the insurance companies are starting to redefine the weight groups; and we seem to be becoming more and more accepting of large people. It's almost the polar opposite of where we were in the '60s." That is, when we weren't so obese.

There are, of course, good and rational reasons to expand the clothing choices available to young people. Youth is a time of great changes in body size and shape; sometimes outsize garments are not a matter of style but of necessity. It is also a time when vulnerable egos can become warped by the inevitable teasing that comes with being overweight or obese. Having stylish clothes like everyone else can alleviate some of that social strain.

But we would be fooling ourselves if, as a culture, we came to believe that such accommodations come without a price, and perhaps a sizable one. Science, history, and common sense all hold that physical reminders of one's excess girth are critical when it comes to controlling further weight gain. One of the first things that experts in the science of weight loss recommend to patients who have lost weight, for example, is to get rid of their old, big-size clothing. The presence of such old clothes simply makes it easier for a person to gain weight; there is something comfortable to go back to. Researchers in the science of satiety — the study of when someone feels full and satisfied with a meal — point to something else. A slight tug at one's waist seems to perform two vital weight-maintaining functions. The first involves the so-called stretch factor, the brain-signaling that occurs when one's stomach is stretched by food intake. Those signals tell the brain when one is satisfied, telegraphing the message that one has eaten enough. A tug at the waist — something absent or diminished by spandex or extra-large-size pants — seems to accentuate that signaling.

Then there is what might be called the theory of the belt, which holds that people will watch and maintain their weight better if they are warned that they are gaining weight by clothing that makes them slightly uncomfortable. Although largely the product of accumulated experience and folk wisdom, there is now a small but important body of science upholding the theory. In the early 1980s, John Garrow, the dean of British obesity studies, looked at the post–weight loss experience of a group of obese patients who had had their jaws wired. Garrow wanted to know if the patients could be prevented from regaining their weight through psychological reminders, or "cognitive thresholds."

Garrow's obese patients who had maintained weight loss had reported that they now wore smaller new clothes. Garrow proposed a test. He fitted half of his subjects with a 2-millimeter-wide nylon waist cord, one tight enough to make a white — but not red — line when seated. A control group was not fitted. The results, he wrote, were "striking differences between the two groups . . . in the weight change after the wires were removed." In the control group, the predictable weight gain had commenced full throttle — at about 1.8 kilograms a month. In the group with the waist cords, however, there was no significant weight gain. Surprisingly, the belt effect seemed to be a lasting one. Five months after the unwiring, the waist cord group had gained significantly less weight than the control group, and the average difference between the two groups "thereafter steadily increased."

Which brings us, full circle, back to our friends at the Olive Garden . . .

About two months after he first heard from Larry, the customer who had complained about how small all the chairs were in his local Olive Garden restaurant, Ron Magruder, the chain's president, received another call. It was Larry again. He was calling in response to a follow-up query from one of Magruder's staff. The staff had been busily making sure that all of the chain's restaurants now had at least three chairs that could accommodate the more amply endowed and had wanted Larry to report what he thought of their efforts.

Well, he *was* happier now. Indeed, Larry's message was entirely conciliatory — even thankful. But it wasn't because of the bigger chairs. It was because of the old small chairs. Largely because of them, Larry explained, he had been spurred to finally confront the extent of his weight problem. Why, in the seven weeks since he had spoken to Magruder, he had lost almost fifty pounds.

That tight little chair — that had been what Larry needed after all.

4

WHY THE CALORIES
STAYED ON OUR BODIES

I F THE 1980S saw the traditional custodians of caloric intake — parents, school, church, and society — go on an extended vacation, the period also witnessed another change. This one took place among those charged with stimulating the nation's physical culture — those whose job it is to promulgate caloric expenditure. The reasons were, as the experts liked to say, "multifactorial," ranging from taxpayer parsimony to denial to outright political dogma. One thing was certain. Increasingly, when it came to public physical fitness — the kind of national venture that JFK so successfully advocated in the early 1960s — the nation was (often literally) out to lunch. Physical fitness? That was an individual pursuit, hardly something on which to waste scarce public resources, let alone actually promote.

As president of the President's Council on Physical Fitness and Sports, Arnold Schwarzenegger had found this out the hard way. Appointed in 1988 by President George Bush, the action movie star had taken up his charge, initially, with all of the fervor and passion one might expect from a man who'd literally remade himself in a cramped California gym only fifteen years before. Spending enormous amounts of time and his own money,

Schwarzenegger had undertaken one of the most ambitious efforts ever at the council: the creation of a national youth fitness consortium. State by state, the Terminator had met with governors and local leaders to found small chapters of "fitness activists," who would then advocate for increased support for state and local physical fitness programs. It was, as Hollywood agents like to say when they get a star to agree to a project, a "way to put a motor in it," the "it" in this case being state-by-state fitness reforms. To highlight the achievements of his state councils, Schwarzenegger had also lobbied for a national fitness day, with colorful festivities planned at state and national parks. On his better days at council meetings Schwarzenegger would even lapse into *gemütlich* reverie, recalling his summers spent at outdoor sporting camps in his native Austria.

But as his term wore on, the *gemütlich* moments grew rarer and rarer, until the Terminator was a notably un-*glücklich* man. In almost every endeavor at the council he had encountered not just resistance to change but often outright insubordination. "I just don't understand and will not accept that it will take you six months to get me the minutes of the last meeting!" he barked at staff members at one board meeting. "What is it here?" There were other troubles. He suspected the American Alliance for Health, Physical Education, Recreation and Dance (AAHPERD), which the council paid to promote its famous fitness test, of not doing its job on the information front. And on his notion for a national sports festival he had got nothing but static. As John Cates, Schwarzenegger's PR adviser at the time, recalls, "We had thirteen lawyers telling us why we could not have a Great American Workout! The Forest Service people moaned about having so many people tromp around in the bushes. And the Parks people couldn't talk about anything but insurance liability." In other words, Washington, D.C., was treating the Terminator just as it would anyone else.

The last indignity came one day in late 1991. Schwarzenegger had successfully signed up governor after governor in his youth fitness campaign, and had come to Little Rock, Arkansas, he hoped, to sign up one more. As a warm-up he had arranged to address members of the Arkansas state assembly on the issue. The speech had gone well. Later that day he was scheduled to meet with the state's young governor to get him to join the crusade. So Schwarzenegger and his entourage arrived at the governor's suite, and began to . . . wait. And wait. Soon Schwarzenegger, recalls Cates, "was really getting anxious." After an hour or so Deputy Governor Jim Guy Tucker appeared and promised that the governor would be there in "just ten minutes." But ten minutes came and ten minutes went. Much later, and after watching a parade of lesser politicos walk upstairs into the governor's office, Schwarzenegger left. Arkansas and Bill Clinton would be the only blank spot on Arnold's list of gubernatorial fitness czars.

Clinton's snub perfectly mirrored his own generation's feelings about public fitness programs. To them, PE, even when one was thinkin' about tomorrow, was just not that important.

Nowhere was this more apparent than in California, once considered the leader in physical fitness programs. From early on, the cult of the body was codified in the Golden State. In 1866, not long after the former Spanish colony became a state, the new legislature directed all public schools to pay "due attention . . . to such physical exercise for the pupils as may be conducive to health and vigor of the body as well as the mind." In 1917 California became one of only a handful of states to require daily physical fitness education. In 1928 the State Board of Education was one of the first such bodies to require four years of PE for graduation, and for the next three decades, even as many school districts in other states waned in their support for public fitness, California went on extending its requirements to elementary and junior college students. With its predictably endless drills of running and jumping about in the brilliant sunlight, PE became a spartan rite of passage — a warm-up for the various other cults of the body that the typical Californian would inevitably encounter later in life.

Although the conventional history dates the decline of PE in

California to Proposition 13, the law that no one voted for, its origins trace themselves to two forces emerging at least five years prior to passage of the 1978 measure. Both were emblematic of the baby boom, its values, and its priorities. The first was Title 9 of the federal Education Amendments, passed in 1972. These much needed provisions held that "no person . . . shall, on the basis of sex, be excluded from participation in, be denied the benefits [of], or be subjected to discrimination under any education program or activity receiving federal financial assistance." Applied to physical education, where classes had long been conducted separately, and where boys' sports received the majority of support, the law was transformative. A year after its implementation, physical education in California went co-ed. Programs once reserved for boys now opened to girls. To accommodate them, PE staffs were split up and reassigned. And because equal facilities were mandated by the law, existing sports fields, equipment, and locker rooms had to be reapportioned as well. By 1978, when all schools were expected to be in complete compliance with the new law, remarkable progress had been made, with girls finally receiving many of the resources long denied on the basis of gender alone.

The progress came with a cost too. In boom times, those costs might have been absorbed by ever expanding school budgets. But the late 1970s were not exactly booming. Government spending was limited not just by economic trepidation, but by the "small is beautiful" philosophy of the state's brainy new governor, a former Jesuit seminarian named Jerry Brown. Brown was the New Age opposite to his father, Pat, who as governor in the early 1960s had put the government — and its huge budget — center stage in the education field. Now the inclination was to contract. Or, as the younger Brown put it, "to focus resources on small projects that might bring fundamental change." The state legislature began retrenching. In 1976, trying to save money while complying with Title 9, the state allowed individual school districts to exempt juniors and seniors from PE requirements. By 1977 a departmental survey found that almost all public schools had done so. It also reported a dangerous trend: "Staffing has been reduced and teaching methods changed as a direct result of the new programs." Such was the first of a hundred ultimately fatal paper cuts on the corpus of modern PE.

Betty Hennessy, a veteran PE teacher and later adviser to the Los Angeles County Office of Education, noticed the on-the-ground changes almost immediately. Where, in the past, unequal but abundant economic resources had allowed physical education instructors to get equipment and personnel support from district headquarters, now "teachers were on their own." With large classes, and the necessity of getting students in, suited up, and then showered and out the gym door, "the PE teacher became little more than a scorekeeper," she says. To relieve the strain, the state legislature passed a bill allowing non-PE teachers to coach. Although this was a bit like having a PE teacher with no science background tutor kids in chemistry, no one, at least at the state level, seemed to notice. By 1980 another Department of Education survey reported that only half of juniors and seniors were taking PE, and that while many schools were "successfully" implementing Title 9, "about 40 percent of schools . . . perceive that it has caused program quality to decline."

The second pre–Proposition 13 trend at work was more personal: the so-called fitness boom of the '70s. Originating in the popularity of aerobics — long, slow running, mainly — and its various health benefits, personal fitness had been taken up passionately by many California adults. The rise of private gyms and celebrity exercise videos was a natural outgrowth. But unlike the old PE, where group participation and peak performance were goals, the underlying premises of the new fitness boom were individualistic and medical. One exercised for specific ends. Many were, of course, purely cosmetic ends. Others were health-based — one exercised to "reduce health risks," or to "feel better about oneself." Fitness, the new acolytes believed, was about self-empowerment, about autonomy, about self-definition. It was, like the Reagan revolution it took place within, all about throwing off the old bourgeois liberalism of the past, particularly its idealistic but — *and everyone knew this* — highly unattainable group goals.

John Cates, then on the physical education faculty at the University of California at San Diego, saw the writing on the wall — but the problem, as he saw it, was not the fitness boom, it was the PE establishment itself. He was particularly frustrated by organizations like the American Alliance for Health, Physical Education, Recreation and Dance (AAHPERD). "We as physical educators were not savvy enough to deal with the change politically," he says. "We had numbers and results, tied to reducing absenteeism and all that, but that case was never marshaled. We were not politically savvy people. I mean, Jane Fonda? Richard Simmons? Give me a break. What a joke. We — AAHPERD — could have made those [fitness] tapes. But the leadership said, no, let other people do it."

With public fitness now seriously endangered, the effects of Proposition 13 cut ever deeper. Overnight the new law sliced $6.8 billion from the state budget. Even with remedial legislation meant to soften Proposition 13's short-term impact, that meant a 25 percent reduction in the schools' share of taxes. Local school boards were now charged with making do. That usually meant making more cuts. By 1980 average PE class sizes had doubled. The percentage of seniors taking PE dipped again, to 43 percent. Enrollment in sports teams dropped in 88 percent of schools, and almost half of all schools eliminated at least one team entirely. In 1983 the legislature codified what had been a reality for nearly half a decade: Students now had to pass only two years of physical education. To this there was little parental opposition.

Which was understandable. For one, many boomers did not exactly harbor the fondest memories of PE, California style. Many recalled it as a time, perhaps the last, when they were unfavorably compared to other people — as in the time they were the last to be chosen to play on the popular kids' team, or the time when, flagging under the scorching sun, they had pooped out only halfway through the calisthenics, or the time they had clearly not won the Presidential Fitness Award, despite really trying at the pull-up bar. No, that wasn't for their child.

And fitness wasn't an important task for schools to perform anyway, was it? After all, there were more important priorities, especially in a nation that had now fallen behind Japan in productivity growth and job creation. Such was the general sentiment, especially after the 1983 report "A Nation at Risk." The study, which emphasized American children's lack of adequate science and math training and its impact on economic opportunity, had become a mantra for the back to basics movement, and in California (and, eventually, around the nation) that had meant anything but physical education. As a 1984 study by the California Department of Education concluded, "In a time of financial strain, declining academic test scores and strong pressure to go 'back to basics,' local school boards appear to have decided to reduce physical education. . . . PE teachers, budgets, enrollment and class size have been sacrificed in favor of 'higher' priorities." The sentiment was clearly not limited to the Golden State. By decade's end, Illinois was the only state to require daily physical fitness education.

What fitness opportunities remained for children grew increasingly class-based. In the nation's more affluent suburbs, where private gym membership by adults had been soaring, a new force emerged: sports clubs for children. Modeled in part on the old Pop Warner and Little League programs of the 1950s, the new clubs, most notably soccer, added a new twist: the notion that "everyone plays." To the boomer parent, psychically singed by the old PE, this was the place for Junior. The new soccer leagues were driven by the enlightened founders and executives of the American Youth Soccer Organization, or AYSO. Founded at an impromptu get-together at the Beverly Hilton in West Los Angeles, AYSO grew by leaps and bounds during the 1980s; between 1974 and 1989 membership increased from 35,000 to

500,000. Because it was essentially driven by parents who had the free time to cart kids to twice-weekly sessions, and who also had the free time to "volunteer" to referee and coach, AYSO was "essentially a suburban movement," as Lollie Keyes, its current communications director, says. "It really wasn't until later that we focused and found the support for inner-city leagues."

The same could be said for almost every other category of youth sports, or, for that matter, for any other opportunity to play — period: Wherever a chance to freely expend calories appeared, it was likely to be contingent upon parental time and money. Or parental residence: Parks and streets tended to be safer in suburbs. And inner cities, increasingly filled with less politically savvy new immigrants, were often shortchanged in parks and recreation spending, not to mention adequate neighborhood policing. All of this was reflected in a 1999 survey by the Daniel Yankelovich consultancy, citing lack of sidewalks and unsafe neighborhoods as "major barriers to fitness." The new unspoken truth was simple: In America, fitness was to be purchased, even if you were a child.

The realities and values of inner-city immigrant life also augured against investments in fitness. In Los Angeles, the Ellis Island of postwar America, new Latin American immigrants proved to be not much different from previous generations of poor immigrants to the United States (save, perhaps, that their proximity to the border rendered them economically more vulnerable to wave upon wave of wage-undermining newcomers). For one, most of their time was spent simply making ends meet, a process often made more draining by a lack of adequate public transportation, affordable housing, and health care. For another, they were not urbanites but rather urban villagers; like the 1950s generation of Italian Americans, they were and are likely to act upon Old World ideas about exercise and health — in essence, the less the better. Studies by University of Pennsylvania epidemiologists under Professor Shiriki Kumanyika, for example, showed that when new immigrants were asked whether rest was more important or better for health than exercise, a large portion "always says yes." The attitude was doubly corrosive: Among immigrant groups at the highest risk for hypertension and diabetes (see chapter 6), many respondents said that exercise "has the potential to do more harm than good."

Such attitudes have been reinforced by a growing knowledge gap about health matters. Consider a 2000 study of 1,929 Americans by American Data Sports Inc. Researchers asked interviewees to agree or disagree with the statement "There are so many conflicting reports, I don't know if exercise is good or bad for me." Thirty-seven percent of those earning under $25,000 agreed, compared with about 14 percent making $50,000 to $75,000 and 12 percent of those making $75,000 or more. Only 46 percent of those with earnings under $25,000 agreed with the statement "I would definitely exercise more if I had the time," compared with 68 percent of those making $50,000 to $75,000 and 67 percent of those making $75,000 and up.

Still, in the 1980s, perhaps more than any other decade, the working class, the middle class, and the affluent shared one inclination: the willingness to use television as their predominant personal leisure time activity. Of course, the observation that Americans watch lots of TV instead of doing other things is hardly novel. But, truth be told, a scientifically rigorous study of that pattern was almost nonexistent until the late 1980s and early 1990s. It was then that Larry Tucker, an exercise physiologist at Brigham Young University, decided to study three interrelated trends. One, that most Americans are sedentary; two, that many feel they do not have the time to exercise; and three, that the average adult watches about four hours of television a day. To find out the extent of that association, and to see if one were causal of the other, Tucker studied the association between TV viewing duration and weekly exercise for 8825 men and women. The results indicated an even stronger association than experts had previously suspected: TV time was strongly and inversely associated with duration of weekly exercise. One example: Among those who reported little or no regular exercise, 9.4 percent viewed less than an hour of TV a day while 33 percent — the largest single group — reported watching three to four hours a day. As Tucker dryly concluded, "Adults who perceive they have too little time to exercise may be able to overcome this problem by watching less television."

But adults were doing more than just kicking back and having a laugh with the *Cheers* gang; more than ever before, they were using the tube as a baby-sitter. It was, after all, an increasingly child-oriented media. With cable expanding and VCR use almost universal, entertainment firms entered the children's "edu-tain-ment" niche with a vengeance, marketing a torrent of children's programs, videos, and games. So did McDonald's, which in 1985 initiated its so-called "tweens" advertising strategy to reach older kids and adolescents (see chapter 5). In the United States, all of this seemed quite natural — in a free market, new needs are created and then new needs are filled. TV was a pragmatic solution to the harried lives that so many new working couples faced. And who was to judge? Only a cynical, and rare, European would be willing to prick the happy bubble, as was the case in 1999, when the French exercise scholar Jean-François Gautier put it this way: "Children are naturally very active, but their parents are restraining them. Children are only allowed to be physically active if adults decide it is appropriate."

More than anything, though, American TV-viewing merged parent and child into one seamless inactivity bubble — a bubble filled with billion-dollar cues to eat, even when one was not hungry. You could argue whether that was morally right or heinously perverted, as did the occasional public TV special. But you couldn't deny the reality as experienced by every American family worth its potato chips. "Kids and dads watching twenty-three to twenty-eight hours a week of TV — that's a lot of sitting," Brigham Young's Larry Tucker observed. "And where there's a lot of sitting, there's lots of snacking."

And a lot of fat children. To find out what the pattern Tucker detected in adults was doing to their offspring, the Centers for

Disease Control in 1994 studied the exercise, television-viewing, and weight gain patterns of 4063 children aged eight to fifteen. The results were stunning (if, in hindsight, predictable). Whether grouped by age, sex, or ethnicity, exercise rates were inversely correlated with TV time, which was in turn positively correlated with increasing body fat percentages. The more TV a child watched the less she exercised and the more likely she was to be either overweight or obese.

What was surprising, though, was the pronounced class and ethnic bent of the numbers. The poor, the black, and the brown not only tended to view more TV than their white counterparts, they also tended to exercise far less. The greatest disparity was between white girls and black girls; where 77.1 percent of the former reported at least three sessions per week of "playing or exercising enough to make me sweat or breathe hard," only 69.4 percent of black girls reported doing the same, with 72.6 percent of Mexican American girls so reporting. When it came to television-viewing, the numbers were even more disquieting. The percentage of white girls who reported watching four or more hours of TV a day was 15.6. The percentage of black girls: 43.1. Of Mexican American girls: 28.3.

Why was that? The CDC surveyed parents. Beyond the usual concerns about time, money, and the "need to rest," one rationale emerged among all parental groups: the concern about crime and how it acted as a barrier to some children becoming more physically active. About 46 percent of all U.S. adults believed that their neighborhoods were unsafe. Among the middle class, such sentiments fueled the growing inclinations to "bubble-wrap" all childhood activity, doubling up on safety precautions and delimiting spontaneous play. And parents in minority neighborhoods were twice as likely as white parents to report that their neighborhoods were dangerous. What the surveyed parents were implying was utterly reasonable: TV-viewing may be bad, but at least my kid won't get shot, molested, kidnapped, or jumped into a gang while doing it.

Yet the greater the TV time, the fatter the child. Cross-index-ing the TV numbers from its 1994 study with skinfold tests (for body fatness) and calculations of body mass index, the CDC found that "boys and girls who watched four or more hours of television per day had the highest skinfold thicknesses and the highest BMIs; conversely, children who watched less than one hour of television a day had the lowest BMIs." This, the study concluded, was a "worrisome trend." No wonder that, between 1966 and 1994, obesity prevalence among youth jumped from 7 percent to 22 percent. Worse, there were huge increases in the percentage of fat children defined as morbidly obese or super-obese — bigger than 95 percent of their peers.

But what did that mean? For one thing, it meant the beginning of a lifetime of medical problems. Study after study had unequivocally indicated that becoming overweight and sedentary as a child or adolescent predicted being obese as an adult. Fat children became fat adults. Moreover, the risks of obesity in adulthood appear to be greater in persons who were overweight in childhood or adolescence. It also meant reduced physical fitness, particularly when it came to cardiovascular fitness. A study by the Amateur Athletic Union of the 1980–1989 period found large increases in the amount of time it took the average child to complete a standardized endurance run. The greatest slowdowns were found in the eight-to-nine-year-old category — exactly the age at which the young are more likely to gain weight anyway.

Numbers, studies, reports, and surveys. By the mid-1990s, they were all saying the same thing: Children were getting fatter, exercising less, eating more (and more often), and watching TV and playing Nintendo in ever greater amounts. Did any of this come as a great shock? No. But what did come as a shock — first in small awarenesses, then in still greater ones — was just how disabled — and just how socially disenfranchised — the young could become from being fat.

In California, the onetime model of physical culture in America, fat abounded. By the late 1990s, only one out of five students in public schools could pass the minimum standards in the state's physical fitness tests. And everywhere — but especially in the Mexican American community — childhood diabetes rates were soaring. So were the rates for a wide variety of other weight-related diseases, among them coronary heart disease, cardiovascular disease, bone disease, and a wide range of endocrine and metabolic disorders. The Spanish-language standard-bearer *La Opinión* often blares: DIABETES, EPIDEMIA EN LATINOS!

There were other, less predictable consequences too. A growing number of Latino children were showing up at their school nurse's office, either for their daily shot of insulin or for a number of other blood sugar regulating medications — so many that the L.A. school administration tried to talk the nurses into letting school secretaries administer the doses in the nurses' absence. (The nurses said no.) There were the victims of the newest form of childhood cruelty — the fat kids who would end up as the target of the daily dodgeball game, wherein balls were hurled so hard as to cause black eyes and bruised midsections, not to mention deep cuts in self-esteem.

And there were the changes occurring outside of school. Strange, weird, tragicomic changes. One of them was taking place in the sport of surfing, long the hallmark of the state's international image as a kingdom of perfect bodies. The change dawned on Steve Pezman, the longtime publisher of *Surfing* magazine, one summer day in the late 1980s. Pezman had headed out to Santa Monica Beach, the most popular of L.A.'s beaches and the destination for thousands of downtown and east side families every weekend. As was his custom, when he got there he sat down and took in the scene. Out on the ocean bobbed the usual lineup of young men and women, waiting for the best wave. They were very white, very lean, and, for the most part, blond. Far closer to the beach floated another lineup, also waiting for waves — essentially for the waves that had been too small or too unformed for the blond kids farther out. The young people in this lineup were very brown and, more often than not, rounder than their white counterparts.

As Pezman sat and watched, he realized what he was really seeing. One, that those in the group closer to shore were not just a little chubby, but downright fat. The other thing he noticed was that many of them could not — or did not — swim very well. Instead, they relied heavily on what had become a standard piece of equipment: the surf leash. The leash attaches the board to the surfer's ankle, so as to prevent the board from getting away after a wipeout and causing the surfer to have to swim after it. Wow, Pezman thought. "Not only had the sport segregated itself according to ability, like any other sport," he recalls. "But it had also segregated itself by body type and by reliance on a laborsaving technology. Unfit surfers! *Fat* surfers!

"Who would have thought?"

Who would have thought? Well, for one, the National Institutes of Health, which had, between 1977 and 1985, issued not one, not two, but three warnings about obesity and its unhealthful effects on both children and adults. To each of these the nation had yawned. *Fortune* magazine, in a typical screed, proclaimed that the real problem was not obesity but, rather, the NIH, which it alleged was using the issue as yet one more way for the government to intrude into "private" affairs. What could one do about such a problem anyway? And who might do it?

More than any one organization, the President's Council on Physical Fitness and Sports might. Founded in 1958 by President Dwight D. Eisenhower after a series of reports detailed the poor fitness of many American troops, the council had long occupied the national bully pulpit on all things PE. Under JFK, it had even asserted a hold on popular culture. Kennedy himself took a leading role in the issue, making much publicized fifty-mile hikes and writing articles on the subject for such popular magazines as *Life* and *Look*. At its core, fitness was to Kennedy a matter of national survival, both literally — a number of studies had shown that Soviet boys had pulled far ahead of American boys in many tests of strength and agility — and metaphorically. "All of us must consider our own responsibilities for the physical vigor of our children and of the young men and women of our communities," he once wrote. "We do not want our children to become a nation of spectators. Rather, we want each of them to be a participant in the vigorous life."

To motivate the nation, the council had turned to the tools of the newly emerging complex of public relations specialists, sports celebrities, and Madison Avenue survey takers. There were specialized fitness magazines for girls (*Vim*) and boys (*Vigor*). There was a council theme song, by *Music Man* composer Meredith Willson; its refrain was "Go You Chicken Fat Go!" It became a national hit. There was the council's charismatic chairman, the baseball great "Stan the Man" Musial. And there were the tests — those annual rites of pull-ups, sit-ups, shuttle runs, and long jumps so loved (or dreaded) by schoolchildren from Sacramento to Poughkeepsie.

All of this seemed to work — or at least to give the impression that it did. In a 1965 survey entitled "Closing the Muscle Gap," Musial wrote: "In 1958 the average 15-year-old American boy could run 600 yards in 2 minutes 19 seconds and do 45 sit-ups. Today's average 15-year-old can run 600 yards in 2 minutes and do 73 sit-ups." Although academics might quibble with the basis of such testing, few could argue with the basic upbeat message, not to mention the council's overall mission. Here were the denizens of Camelot, doing jumping jacks in the sun.

By 1985, however, when it confronted the results of its third national survey, the council had evolved into a more complicated beast. At its head sat its celebrity chairman, the football coach George Allen. A longtime friend of Republican presidents, Allen was obsessed with one idea: the creation of a national academy of fitness. Characteristically, he had thrown all of his energy, charm, and connections into the task, and spent most of his time on the road, raising funds, locating possible sites for the campus, and enlisting old gridiron buddies in the cause.

This left the running of the council increasingly to its executive director, a former San Diego PE teacher and fitness expert named Ash Hayes. Tall, rangy, and physically striking, Hayes was the embodiment of the postwar California fitness buff. Born and raised in Iowa, he had moved to California after a stint in the army during World War II. "My parents had moved there, and once I saw no one ever shoveled snow there, I decided to get my BA in San Diego," he recalled. "I turned into a beach lover." And a fitness lover. As an administrator in the San Diego school district, Hayes had found himself drawn to the growing field of physical fitness. He began to teach the subject. Then to coach. "The need for fitness was always very clear to me, really instinctive," he says. "Even as an undergraduate and as a young farmer and soldier before that, everything told me that the body was designed to be physically active. It was common sense." By 1981 Hayes was head of the health and physical education department of the San Diego City School District, and president of a number of national fitness and sports organizations.

By then he was also a regular in California Republican party politics. So when Casey Conrad, a longtime GOP activist friend and then the council's executive director, called on him for assistance, Hayes said yes. He first served as the council's state coordinator, then as co-director. In 1985 Conrad retired. Hayes assumed the directorship.

He also assumed a headache. Just that year the council had released its third national fitness survey. As with the one it had done in 1975, results were lackluster. Studying the fitness abilities of eighteen thousand American boys and girls, the survey had concluded not only that there had been little general improvement in overall fitness levels, but that there also had been slippage, particularly among young girls. About 50 percent of them (compared to 30 percent of boys) could not run a mile in fewer than ten minutes. The same held true of other test items, from the 50-yard dash to the flexed arm hang. Among girls in particular, the rate of improvement was flat, with some declines in individual age group performance.

But for Hayes, that wasn't the worst of it. At almost the same time the results of a parallel study were published, this one conducted by the U.S. Public Health Service. The report looked at the ability of 8800 students to perform rigorous physical tests designed to assess overall health and fitness. The results showed that about half of American children were not getting enough exercise to develop healthy hearts and lungs. Even more alarming was what the service found out about fatness and American youth. Median skinfold sums were 2 to 3 millimeters thicker than a sample taken by the PHS in the mid-1960s. Kids were getting fatter.

Yet if his mission was growing larger by the day, Hayes's resources were shrinking, partly from Reagan-era budget cuts, partly from pure lack of interest by other arms of government. "My total budget was $1.5 million," Hayes recalls. "That, basically, was zero. We were constantly with our hat in hand, trying to find corporate sponsors for various projects." Some of those sponsors eventually included such unlikely partners as 7-Up and McDonald's, "but we never thought of that as a conflict of interest, because we never let them use the council seal in their advertising."

Despite the lack of resources, when it came to communicating the issue of fitness, the council already owned one potent weapon: its annual Presidential Fitness Awards and the tests that went with them. True, there were better, more scientific assessments of fitness. But none had the standing or reach into the average home and school in quite the way that the council's did. By 1985 the award had been won by some 8 million American children.

Since its inception, the test had been administered by the American Alliance for Health, Physical Education, Recreation and Dance (AAHPERD), the nation's leading organization of fitness professionals. It had been designed at a meeting of its research council in February 1957, when members — responding to Eisenhower's plea to develop some way to measure American youth's declining fitness level — came up with eight tests. These were the pull-up (for boys), modified pull-ups (for girls), sit-ups, the standing broad jump, the shuttle run, the 50-yard dash, the softball throw, and the 600-yard run. Over the next decade there would be minor tweaks to the regimen; in 1964 the modified pull-up for girls was replaced by the flexed arm hang, the softball throw was eliminated, and modified sit-ups (with flexed knees) were substituted for the conventional straight-legged ones.

But by and large the test proved amazingly durable. By 1975 some 65 million pupils had been tested. The president's council adopted the test as a basis for its own Presidential Fitness Award, given to any child who scored in the top 15 percent of his or her age group. It awarded a lucrative contract to AAHPERD to conduct the test. To recoup some of its costs, the council sold its award patches to individual school districts.

Yet even within AAHPERD, the test was controversial. Many of its own members had argued that pull-ups and 50-yard dashes and standing broad jumps had little to do with fitness and everything to do with measuring performance. This, they argued, was because the battery had been designed with largely military concerns in mind. In that context, the pull-up made sense — every soldier ought to be able to pull himself out of a foxhole. So did the broad jump, the flexed arm hang, the softball throw, and the 50-yard dash. A good soldier should be able to jump quickly out of harm's way, lob a grenade, hang from a window, or sprint toward the engagement line.

But what did those abilities have to do with fitness for everyday life? For two decades AAHPERD, despite the rising chorus of its own members, sidestepped the question, at least when it came to the tests for the council's Presidential Fitness Awards. If this was what the client wanted, that is what they would give the client. Such was the thinking until two trends came to undo it.

The first was the ascendance of aerobic exercise — jogging, as experienced by most Americans of the 1970s. The concept had been popularized by Kenneth Cooper, a former military physician who, after almost dying of a heart attack, had restored himself to top condition through what he liked to call "LSD — long slow distance" running. At the core of Cooper's exercise prescription — which he detailed in his 1968 bestseller *Aerobics* — was one key fact: that improvements in cardiovascular abilities — the ability to use and expend oxygen — came mainly from moderate increases in energy expenditure. In the past, conventional wisdom had held just the opposite. The old notion was that one would have to raise one's "Vmax2" — deciliters of oxygen expended per kilogram of body weight — to over 60 in order to force the body and its muscles to get stronger and to endure more. Using a treadmill, Cooper had demonstrated that such "training effects" actually happened at a much lower level of exercise, at, say, a Vmax2 of 40. In other words, it was better (and more efficient) to jog slowly for a half-hour than to run swiftly for ten minutes. Cooper also showed that body composition, specifically percentage of fat, played a big role in cardiovascular health, regardless of whether or not you could sprint 50 yards or jump 8 feet. In this light AAHPERD's — and the council's — preference for things like 600-yard runs looked highly unscientific, if not downright archaic.

The second force was the rise of a new generation of exercise physiologists, scientists who study exactly how the body responds to various forms of physical activity. Of these men and women, none was more aggressive — and intellectually pugnacious — than Charles "Chuck" Corbin. A Cooper protégé and a professor at Arizona State University, Corbin had long harbored reservations about the AAHPERD fitness test. As a young PE teacher he had administered it himself, year after year, only to observe something that he found deeply disquieting. "Basically, the same kids won it year after year," he recalls. "And eventually some of us began to say, 'Hey, wait a minute — the so-called fit kids under this test are the ones who already got the award patch, and the kids who aren't fit under this test, well, they just give up.' So kids came to hate PE. I became convinced that this was a bad thing — I saw that they grew up to be parents who hated PE too." Then, in a series of studies conducted with his co-author Bob

Pangrazi, also of ASU, Corbin was able to show that almost every item on the AAHPERD test battery correlated not with one's fitness levels, but with one's hereditary and environmental advantages. Moreover, the decades-long notion that only children who tested better than 85 percent of their peers deserved an achievement award didn't make scientific sense either. Corbin and Pangrazi saw significant fitness improvements in those who scored as low as the 50th percentile. Combined with Cooper's growing body of work documenting the importance of longer distances run more slowly, a new consensus began to emerge among younger AAHPERD members. "Many of us started to say, 'Why is activity important? What kinds of activity are important to adulthood that we were not teaching in schools?' We started to say, 'Hey, what's important to lifelong fitness? What things really made a difference?' We were saying that not everybody could be a sports star. And that, to be candid, was very counter to the ideals of the founders [of the council], who all thought that every kid would be able to get into the 85th percentile."

By 1980 Corbin and Pangrazi had convinced AAHPERD to develop a new test, this one designed to assess health-related fitness skills. The new one was Corbin and Cooper, distilled. Gone was almost every item on the traditional test. Instead, there were distance runs (one for nine minutes, one for twelve minutes, and one for the mile) for cardiovascular health, a sit-and-reach test to measure flexibility, modified sit-ups for trunk strength, and, truly radical, skinfold measurements for body fatness. Developed with Cooper at his Dallas Texas Institute, the new test would be called the "Fitnessgram."

Right away, the new test rankled the old-timers, who viewed it as a form of "dumbing down." As Hayes saw it, "if you ask less of people you will always get less from people — everything in my background told me that. Why was a pull-up so important? Ask any soldier who had to pull himself out of a foxhole, or any fireman who had to hang from the window of a burning building." John Cates, then an assistant to George Allen, also worried about the dumbing-down effect, but also says, "There was a whole self-esteem issue here, and not just of the variety of 'making it easier' so kids don't feel bad about not getting an award. The financial cutbacks in the schools had also done something else to PE classes — it forced very dissimilar kids, kids of very different physical abilities, into one class, where comparisons were inevitable." He adds: "But one thing was clear: The kids were getting worse and worse. Do you water this down? Do you lower standards or do you keep the old ones and possibly stigmatize some kids?" To this Corbin again responded with new data that showed — convincingly — that far from inspiring children to work harder, the old standards simply turned them off to exercise altogether. "The basic response of most kids was 'why bother?'"

After a few years, it was clear that the new test was becoming troublesome in another way: It began to confuse school districts, which could not distinguish it from the more traditional council test. In effect, AAHPERD had created a competitor to one of its most important clients.

To reconcile the two tests, AAHPERD and the council set up an advisory committee. For three years those favoring a health-based test battled over one key bone of contention: the council's insistence on maintaining the 85th percentile. Though it was something both sides felt deeply about, the science clearly favored the reformers. And so, by 1986, as the annual AAHPERD conference approached, the two groups reached for a consensus: In the new test there would be elements from both the old test and the new. They also agreed to consider a new awards scheme — one, as Corbin saw it, "that was based on science, and that rewarded process and improvement rather than the end product."

Then, just as both groups prepared to announce the new test, the council, led by Hayes, threw up a new barrier: the body composition test. It was, he said, "inappropriate." It might hurt kids' feelings. And it might make parents mad that someone was touching their child. Anyway, Hayes said, the council "wasn't ever in the business of making weight an issue."

But for the council, such opposition to the "weight issue" *was* something new. Ever since its founding, body weight had been a key element of its agenda. The council's theme song, after all, had been quite explicit about the goal of exercise — "Go You Chicken Fat Go!" In the 1970s the council had further focused on the issue of body weight and health by sponsoring a highly visible ad campaign, designed by Young and Rubicam and placed in leading general interest magazines. In one ad depicting a chubby boy eating an ice cream and surrounded by TVs, radios, telescopes, and model airplanes — symbols of sedentary behavior — the copy read: "We're so overdeveloped we're underdeveloped." Another showed a giant marshmallow and declared "Hey kid! If you see yourself in this picture, you need help," only to go on to say, "There's a little marshmallow in all of us. A little blob. A little cream puff. A little jelly belly." Another simply proclaimed: "There's no such thing as stylishly stout."

Although these were certainly not the way to approach the issue now, the reformers, led by Cooper and Corbin, insisted that weight was now even more relevant to health. There was a direct and well-documented link between excess body fat and all manner of heart disease, not to mention various bone and endocrine disorders. Knowing one's body composition was key to knowing how healthy one was and what one had to do to become healthier. "As we saw it — and as we presented it — body fat testing was no different than, say, getting a mammogram or a prostate exam," Corbin recalls. "What test isn't a little embarrassing?"

To this Hayes's allies countered with what was — for them, at least — an unlikely refrain. Putting too much emphasis on body weight, they said, could inadvertently promote anorexia. In an era when the disease had become a talk show staple, with fashion advertising the leading enemy, it was an emotional and effective debate tactic. But it was also scientifically dubious. Even the most generous epidemiological estimates put anorexia far down on the list of mainstream teenage woes.

By April 1986, when the two sides were to meet at the AAHPERD annual meeting, what was once a relatively collegial process had broken down. The council and its supporters had come out against the skinfold test and for inclusion of the shuttle run — two decisions the reformers could not abide. "We were basically shut out," Corbin recalls. "The council showed up and began handing out copies of the printed test, with our name on it! We never got a chance to present the new test." Cooper was furious. Learning of the shutout, he walked out of the conference, taking the Fitnessgram with him. As Corbin saw it: "We blew a great chance to put parents on notice that body composition should be one thing they ought to consider when they assess their kids' health."

And they had blown it during a decade when the caloric environment for children was growing ever more toxic.

Hayes and the old guard may have been wrong about the body fat test, but on the subject of health-based exercise prescriptions they may have been more on target than many in today's fitness establishment would like to admit. If their fear that expecting less from children would lead to diminished caloric expenditure — in effect a tacit endorsement of sloth — such a fear was arguably even more justified when it came to a new set of exercise recommendations for adults that began appearing in the early 1990s, at exactly the time when sedentary behavior was at an all-time high and supersized portions and snacking became the norm.

To understand how radical the new recommendations were, consider what had been the standard "exercise Rx" prior to the 1990s. Until then, almost every organization that was in the business of making public health recommendations agreed on several things. One, that exercise should consist of sustained activity — "15–60 minutes of continuous aerobic activity," at least three to five days a week, as the American College of Sports Medicine (ACSM) put it in its formal 1978 position paper. Implicit in this was a key assumption: that the more one exercised, the more benefits one got from that exercise. This the experts called the "dose-response effect." The second point of accord related to exercise intensity. To be effective, exercise should be moderate to vigorous, with a Vmax2 — maximum oxygen uptake — of 50 to 85, with a preference for the upper end. As J. N. Morris, the reigning dean of exercise physiology, put it in 1980, "Adequate exercise means vigorous exercise."

But all through the 1980s, exercise levels among adults, which had been on the rise since the 1960s, began to plateau, then to fall. Experts attributed this to the modern lifestyle. Americans were working more hours, spending more time commuting, and, increasingly, working jobs that were not "sweat-friendly." The new American worker toiled not in a factory or even a giant corporation, but, rather, in the rising field of professional services. They had to dress nicely, or at least semi-nicely. They hardly had the time to change, exercise, shower, and get back to their desks at lunchtime. Or so the experts said.

Of course, there was another way to look at the American worker, and that was as a person with an increasingly flexible, project-oriented job. Certainly the personal computer had created vast new groups of people who telecommuted, worked from home, or — especially in the enterprising 1980s, when new business formation was at an all-time high — actually struck out on their own. One thing was certain: The typical American worker still had time for four hours of television every night.

Nevertheless, confronted with declining exercise numbers and alarming rates of cardiovascular disease, public health officials felt that something had to be done about the traditional exercise recommendations. Studies had shown that adults, like children, reacted badly to high expectations. In this view, the plateauing of their exercise rates was one big "why bother?" As in the field of physical education, a new consensus emerged among America's leading adult exercise scholars. It was time to "be more realistic" about exercise prescriptions.

Like Cooper and Corbin, these reformers — many of them using data from Cooper's own studies of adults who came to his clinic — had new science on their side. Big studies were showing two interesting trends that supported their views. One, that moderate, not vigorous, activity was key to reducing major health risks like heart attack and stroke. And two, that *total accumulated* caloric expenditure was just as good as sustained continuous exercise when it came to reducing risk of heart attack, stroke, hypertension, and a wide range of chronic diseases. On both these accounts, the two most important studies — one of Harvard alumni, the other of white business executives who had come to Cooper's Aerobics Institute for fitness consultation — agreed.

In the Harvard study, men who had the highest total number of minutes of daily activity — walking to work, taking the stairs instead of the elevator, participating in light sports like bowling and gardening — also tended to have the lowest rates of these diseases. (In fact — and this would tickle many a fat boy who hated sports in school — ex–varsity athletes retained a lower-risk profile only if they maintained a high physical activity rate as an adult.) From the point of view of public policy — and of people who wanted a more palatable exercise prescription — the Harvard study provided two key debating points. The first was this: The biggest improvements in health risk reduction occurred not at the higher end of the activity curve, but at the lower — in other words, not among alums who expended, say, 5000 calories a week, but among those who exercised off 1000 calories a week. (Those who expended fewer than 500 calories a week still carried the highest risk.) The second observation was quiet, but, in a way, revolutionary. In the past experts had believed that exercise and fitness were linked in a dose-response effect — more exercise meant more fitness — but the Harvard study showed a leveling-off effect. After about 2500 calories of activity per week, the reduction in risk from heart attack didn't continue to fall. "If there is a causal relationship," its authors concluded, "the figure depicts a plateau of benefit rather than a continuing gradient benefit." If you are trying to reduce your risk of heart attack — and only that — expending more than 2500 calories a week on moderate exercise is a waste of time. In fact, if you are sedentary, you can reduce risk with much less exercise than you thought you could. As the Stanford cardiology professor Robert DeBusk would conclude in a separate 1990 paper in the influential *American Journal of Cardiology:* "High intensity exercise affords little additional benefit."

The Cooper studies provided the reformers with more ammo. Looking at the treadmill tests of 13,000 largely upper-middle-class white men and women, researchers were able to pinpoint exactly where the greatest health benefits, or risk reductions, occurred. Once again, it was at the low end. People who exercised just a little more than people who didn't exercise at all got a bigger percentage reduction in health risks than did people who were already exercising moderately and who then began exercising vigorously. "A brisk walk of 30–60 minutes a day will be sufficient," the authors concluded.

A brisk walk of 30 to 60 minutes a day, however, was still challenging to most Americans. But now two key terms — moderate and cumulative — took on a life of their own. Increasingly, as medical and professional organizations revised their standards to "be more realistic," and as the government began funding studies of "user-friendly" (read: easier) exercise prescriptions, such organizations looked not to the initial recommendations of the Harvard and Cooper authors. Instead, they looked to the key revelations of those studies — or, rather, to their own institutional interpretation of those revelations.

The American Heart Association was the first to jump on the bandwagon. In a lengthy 1990 special report, it downplayed its old recommendations of 2000+ calories a week and instead called for a minimum of "700 calories a week on three or more nonconsecutive days." Walking, the authors advised, "appears to be just as beneficial as more vigorous activities." And more: "Some benefit is apparently derived from as little as 20 minutes of low-intensity exercise three times a week." They then went out of their way to denigrate more vigorous activity, saying simply that "there is no evidence of a health benefit at more than 2000 calories a week."

This was a slightly different line than the evidence suggested, but now intellectual parricide — not scientific precision — drove the effort. Morris be damned. Vigor be damned. Even the authors of the Cooper and Harvard studies joined in, in 1992 proclaiming that "the response to exercise training is primarily, if not exclusively, dependent upon the total energy expended in exercise and not intensity."

Enter now the American College of Sports Medicine. For years it had cagily viewed the reform movement, only slowly lowering its Vmax2 recommendations from 70 to 50 in 1986, and then to 40–60 in 1991. During that time the ACSM's composition had changed; more and more of its most vocal members were not people primarily concerned with exercise as a way to better one's performance in everyday life — the foxhole-digging, window-hanging cadres of the postwar period — but rather scholars who were mainly interested in reducing the risk of chronic diseases, particularly heart disease. In 1993 they seized control, and in a bold and highly publicized paper issued a new exercise manifesto. Backed by the CDC, they issued the following statement: "Every American adult should accumulate 30 minutes or more of moderate intensity physical activity over the course of most days of the week . . . Activities that can contribute to the 30-minute total include walking upstairs (instead of taking the elevator), gardening, raking leaves, dancing, and walking part or all of the way to or from work . . . One specific way is to walk two miles briskly."

This, of course, was a far cry from Morris's old "adequate exercise means vigorous exercise." But it was also a long trek from the reformers' original recommendation of 30 to 60 minutes a day of brisk walking. And it hardly grew from a sense of scientific certainty. After all, only six months before, one of the CDC-ACSM panel's most influential members, Stanford's Ralph Paffenbarger, Jr., had concluded that "what kinds of physical activity should be prescribed, how much, how intense, and for whom *if optimal health and longevity are to be achieved* [emphasis mine] remain unanswered questions that require further clarification."

What had happened? For one, the CDC, as one panel member recalls, "was under tremendous pressure to come up with more palatable recommendations." Behind this was the surgeon general's own Healthy People 2000 Initiative, which had set ambitious public health goals but had little in the way to measure any progress toward such goals. A new set of recommendations was critical to the initiative's success, or at least its bureaucratic success. If one defined minimum fitness too high — if one set the bar so as automatically to make the majority of Americans appear too sedentary — how could there be even the possibility of success by millennium's end, when the surgeon general hoped to have dramatically changed American health habits?

The other *force majeure* lay in the new consensus among the ACSM majority. Many of these men and women had spent the better part of their academic lives studying what they called "exercise compliance" — how, why, and under what circumstances people tended to stick with a regimen. Although these studies tended to focus on specific (and often very small) high-risk groups, their conclusions were nearly unanimous: People tended to stick with regimens that they did not see as overly demanding. In short, the issuers of the new doctrine of "moderate, accumulated" activity believed that the average American would react to their new standards with one great "Wow! I can do that!"

When it comes to exercise, however, human beings are, in general, not a very "Wow! I can do that!" bunch. They are, after all, genetically programmed to conserve energy, to find every opportunity they can to . . . sit on their duffs. Moreover, the new recommendations came at a time of unparalleled opportunity both to be sedentary and to consume huge amounts of fatty calories on the cheap. In the early 1990s supersize had met Super Mario with a vengeance; the price of both had dropped so much as to induce price wars.

Considering such a context, two questions seem appropriate. One, was telling people they could get by with less exercise a good idea? And two, was it true, or at least were the assumptions behind the advice true? On both counts, the evidence suggests an answer of no.

One way to gauge the response of the average American to the new guidelines is to look at the way they were presented by the media. True, the media (thank God) do not exactly represent the way the average Jane thinks, but the modern media are nothing if not absolutely addicted to the latest health manifestos. If skepticism about them is not their lot, the media's acceptance is largely based on ignorance and wishful thinking; to paraphrase Mr. Dooley, the newspaper bosses — they like to sit around and eat a Big Mac too.

Consider what they wrote in the aftermath of the 1993 guidelines: "Still don't exercise? No sweat. A little at a time now called enough" (*Chicago Tribune*); "Gym workout? U.S. says walking, gardening will do, too" (*Boston Globe*); "Study says you don't have to sweat fitness routine" (*Los Angeles Times*); "If you can't run for health, a walk will do, experts say" (*New York Times*); and "A walk is as good as a workout" (*Atlanta Constitution*). TV, as usual, trumped print. In one famous piece by a Los Angeles network affiliate, viewers were told that "even seriously hunting for the channel changer can count toward your daily thirty!"

No one can say exactly how the average American interpreted such drivel, but what, given the permissiveness of the overall culture, would be the better bet: that they would use it as an excuse, as a way to get off the hook, or that they would say, "Wow! I can do that"? The point is that no one on the reform committee seems to have understood the way American culture digests *any* form of reduced expectations. In this case, the media had transformed what was once a mere prescription to reduce a lazy man's chance of getting a heart attack into a national prescription for fitness. In the wishful-thinking, reality-denying, boundary-hating world of modern America, this was manna from heaven — a Whopper with cheese from the CDC!

For all of which the reformers can be forgiven. No one, after all, can ever truly gauge what the popular media will do with any given piece of scientific information. Yet science does answer to its own. And in that respect the reformers have much to reconsider.

How wise was it to base a recommendation for all Americans on the experience of the rich? That is, essentially, what both of the key studies were. These populations of lawyers and business executives may have looked much like average Americans; their body weights, rates of various diseases, and dietary patterns may have been not that different from those of a lineman for the telephone company or a data processor for an insurance company. But their total life experiences were very different. What made thirty minutes of accumulated activity a prophylactic against heart disease for the rich — with their already highly buffered existence — would likely, one might surmise, be much more dilute for the middle class, even more so for the poor. This is because when the rich garden, even briskly, they are doing so with all the other health advantages that come with being rich. Their mini-dose of exercise is amplified by socioeconomics. Not so with the middle class, let alone the poor.

And what about moderate exercise over vigorous exercise, or accumulated activity over sustained, and the idea that most benefits accrue at the low end of activity increases? To what degree did those notions hold up? New reviews are increasingly calling them all into question.

Perhaps the most vexing arena of controversy involves what was the most radical part of the new recommendations — the notion that accumulated activity is as beneficial as sustained activity. This was the element of the reform plan that engendered such creative interpretations as "doing a few minutes of housework" or "intensely bowling." In the scientific literature it is known as "fractionalization of physical activity." To date, evidence for such *as an exercise prescription* (rather than as an observation of activity patterns of the rich) rests largely on one single study involving thirty-six subjects. In it, eighteen healthy men completing thirty minutes of exercise training a day were compared with eighteen men completing three daily ten-minute bouts. Both exercised at a moderate rate — at about 65 to 75 percent of their peak treadmill test heart rate. The authors, led by Stanford's Robert F. DeBusk, concluded that "multiple short bouts of moderate intensity exercise training significantly increase peak oxygen intake," thereby implying that multiple rounds were as good as sustained rounds.

But closer reading leaves one wondering about that conclusion. This is because, at each and every point of comparison, the sustained group performed better than the fractionated group. Peak oxygen intake of the sustained group improved by 4.4 points, as opposed to the fractionated group, which improved by only 2.4 points. Adherence to each respective regimen was the same — thus undermining another supposed advantage of the multiple-session doctrine. The sustained group tended to complete its training session more often than did the fractionated group. As the authors themselves stated, "multiple short bouts of exercise increased peak oxygen uptake 57 percent as much as a single long bout." In other words, a bit more than half as much as the sustained group. These were, to be sure, small differences, and it was clear that the fractionated exercisers were getting more benefit than previously thought. But that was a long way from emphasizing, as the authors did, that "high intensity exercise affords little additional benefit."

What about the general notion behind the recommendations — that health benefits of physical activity are linked principally to the total amount of activity performed? Again, the latest data suggest otherwise. In a more recent work, Paffenbarger found that Harvard alumni who took up moderately vigorous sports activity significantly reduced their mortality risk from all causes compared with those who did not engage in such activity. "In contrast," the scholar Paul Williams has noted in a recent *Archives of Internal Medicine* report, which reanalyzed Paffenbarger's data, "increasing the overall daily activity had no significant impact on overall mortality." Intensity trumped total accumulated activity.

Even more recently, Williams, of the Lawrence Berkeley National Laboratory, produced a stunning series of papers that, in toto, undermine every single assumption of the 1993 recommendations. In a study of 8283 male recreational runners, he revived the old, rejected notion of a dose-response effect. As he put it, "Our data suggest that substantial health benefits occur at exercise levels that exceed current minimum guidelines and do not exhibit a point of diminishing return." In July 2000 Williams eviscerated the new doctrine again, this time by performing a meta-analysis of twenty-three fitness studies representing 1,325,004 person-years of follow-up. The result showed that the risks of heart disease decreased linearly with increasing amounts of physical activity — a clear dose-response effect. "Formulating physical activity recommendations on the basis of fitness studies," like the Cooper and Harvard projects, he concluded in the ACSM's own journal, "may inappropriately demote the status of physical fitness as a risk factor *while exaggerating the public health benefits of moderate amounts of physical activity* [Williams's emphasis]."

It was, of course, easy to dismiss a lone voice in the wind, which is how Williams has been greeted by the reformers. But the snickering turned stone serious in mid-2001, when the ACSM published the findings of a symposium on the subject of "dose response issues concerning physical activity and health." Looking at a number of its own studies over the years, the panel found that "overall, there is a consistent inverse dose-response relationship between physical activity and both the incidence and mortality rates from all cardiovascular and coronary heart disease." It also notes that the dose-response relationship held true for prevention of type 2 diabetes, colon cancer, and obesity.

Slowly — and quietly — the reformers have begun to recognize their errors. The ACSM itself recently published a third position statement calling for a larger volume of activity performed at higher intensities than the 1993 statement. An even more recent study, this one on diet, lifestyle, and type 2 diabetes by the Harvard School of Public Health, goes the extra distance as well. Noting that "current strategies have not been very successful, and the prevalence of obesity continues to increase," the study repeatedly clarifies and amplifies what is meant by adequate physical activity — "vigorous sports, jogging, brisk walking, heavy gardening, heavy housework — vigorous enough to build up a sweat."

The most recent round of "Dietary Guidelines" meetings also called the conventional wisdom to account. Noting that members of the Weight Registry, the only large database that tracks people who have lost weight and kept it off for three years or more, average 2825 calories of exercise a week, compared with the current 1000-calorie recommendation by the American College of Sports Medicine, one prominent member declared, "Are we being aggressive enough or are we simply setting guidelines that we hope will be more appealing to people who have not been successful?"

Canadian health authorities, which have long followed the U.S. lead, have been bolder; adults, they advise, should get sixty minutes of physical activity every day. Why? Because, as the ACSM's journal put it, "the assumption [is] that most people interpret the public health message in terms of predominantly light intensity activities, thus the necessity to recommend a larger daily volume."

Translation: People are lazy, so it does not pay to give them an out when it comes to exercise. It is better to ask for more — not less.

Yet asking for more has become anathema to health policy makers in the realm of fitness. Consider, for example, the strange story of the nation's weight control guidelines.

The guidelines are promulgated every five years by a small,

elite group of nutrition scholars who meet at the USDA's South Agriculture building on Independence Avenue. There they discuss what might be the government's single most important public health action — issuance of the agency's twice-a-decade "Dietary Guidelines for Americans." With spiffy graphics and a multimillion-dollar publicity budget, the guidelines are supposed to communicate the state of the art in nutritional science and health recommendations. Functionally, the guidelines also serve as something else. Almost shamanically they act as the national conscience on matters of food, exercise, and weight control. Their incessant repetition on TV, on radio, in schools, and in popular fitness forums sets the mood for the nation on such issues, ratcheting up and down the guilt levels on various dietary behaviors.

By 1990 the weight control recommendations of the Dietary Guidelines Committee had already been loosened once. In 1980 the guidelines had advised Americans to "maintain an ideal weight" — a clear, unequivocal message that anyone who could read one of those omnipresent weight-for-height charts could understand. By 1985, in the middle of the supersize revolution, the advice was altered to the more vague "maintain a desirable weight," the better not to impose unrealistic goals upon an increasingly touchy populace. In 1990, even as obesity rates spiraled upward, the committee wanted not only to loosen the weight guidelines again, it also wanted to do something it had never done before. It wanted to tell Americans that it was okay to gain significant amounts of weight as they got older.

The impetus had come from Dr. Reubin Andres, a remarkable man with a peculiar agenda. The chief of the metabolism section of the National Institute on Aging, Andres had a long and deep track record in the area of gerontology, diabetes research, and public health policy. (By the mid-1990s he would also enter the annals of medical history as the inventor of the euglycemic clamp, to date the best way to measure insulin secretion and sensitivity in human beings.) In the 1980s Andres had become obsessed with the issue of weight guidelines for the elderly. For four decades, he argued, the nation had hewn to an unnecessarily strict weight-for-height chart set down by the Metropolitan Life Insurance Company. Those standards, he said, were not only unrealistic but also unscientific; they reflected only the experience of people who could afford life insurance, a largely white, affluent, and middle-aged cohort that no longer represented the increasingly diverse country.

To prove his point, Andres performed a statistical reanalysis of what was then Metropolitan Life's most recent data, published in 1979. Also known as the Build Study, the data had become the basis for new weight-for-height recommendations issued in 1983. Andres turned a new lens on the data: What if one broke the data up into age groupings, then asked, essentially, "At what weight-for-height ranges does minimum mortality occur in each age bracket?" Andres and a few colleagues used the question to guide a reworking of the Met Life numbers. They came up with a surprising revelation. As Andres read the revised data, the Metropolitan recommendations were "too low." It was better — that is, less risky — to be fatter — up to fifteen pounds fatter — once one turned forty. This was because "the Metropolitan Life tables have erred, apparently in an effort to simplify the weight recommendations, by not entering age as a variable."

Andres then assessed twenty-three weight studies of other populations, ranging from Japanese men in Hawaii to American Indians. "We compared the body mass indices associated with the lowest mortality from these studies with the body mass indices of the Metropolitan tables," he wrote. Again, the results seemed revolutionary. Higher weights were associated with lower rates of death, particularly among persons over age forty. The recommended weights were thus "too restrictive." A forty-year-old could thus be up to 20 percent fatter than previously thought and still be at minimum added risk from weight-related death. In December 1985 Andres published his findings in the prestigious *Annals of Internal Medicine*. He then embarked on an extensive lobbying effort to change the USDA's weight guidelines, speaking frequently at gatherings of public health experts, advocates for the elderly, and various special-interest groups.

Andres was certainly on to *something*. The goal of crafting weight guidelines that more closely reflect America's racial and ethnic diversity was a righteous one. For decades, even conservative scholars of actuarial data knew that their subject pool, like Cooper's data on rich executive exercisers, was unrepresentative of the national experience. The problem was getting good data on those populations — data that were both statistically *and* medically sound. Unfortunately, Andres had erred on both those counts — erred badly. Yet for two years he went unchallenged, his conclusions slowly but surely taking hold in the national consciousness. Anti-diet and fat rights groups cited him regularly in discussions of why being fat wasn't really a problem. Feminists concerned about anorexia took heart in the notion that the good fight was not against fat but against "unrealistic leanness." It was okay to gain weight.

Then in 1987 four scholars from Harvard University's School of Public Health, led by Walter Willett and Meir Stampfer, dropped a bomb on Andres's research. Trained in epidemiology as well as diabetes and obesity, the quartet closely examined twenty-five of the major prospective studies on body weight and longevity, including the 1979 Metropolitan Life Build Study, the cornerstone of Andres's work. If Andres had been surprised by his reworking of the numbers, the Harvardites were downright frightened by their own. In each and every study they found biases that were so severe and substantial that "failure to address any one issue will lead to an underestimate of excess mortality associated with being overweight." The biases led, they concluded in the *Journal of the American Medical Association,* to a "systematic underestimate of the impact of obesity on premature mortality." It was not okay to gain weight as one aged.

These were fighting words. But Willett and Stampfer had done their homework. Perhaps the most egregious flaw in most of the studies was their authors' failure to control for cigarette smoking, which is an independent risk factor that is more prevalent among the lean than the fat. (Smoking inhibits caloric intake and increases metabolic rates and energy expenditure.) Thus, to get an accurate picture of the added risk of premature death from excess weight, one must "deduct" the effect of smoking. If the statistician does not do this, Willett and Stampfer argued, one comes away with an artificially high mortality rate in lean subjects. That makes being heavier look less risky when it is actually more so.

This was not mere academic nitpicking. Controlling for independent risk factors is a widely accepted — indeed required — protocol in modern epidemiology. Willett and Stampfer had done just that. The results: "After controlling for smoking," they wrote, "the risk of death . . . increased by two percent for each pound of excess weight for ages 50 to 62, and by one percent per extra pound for ages 30 to 49." The same conclusion was reached after reanalyzing an American Cancer Society survey of 750,000 men and women: There was no basis for recommending more lenient weight guidelines. In fact, the numbers suggested just the opposite: Weight guidelines needed to be stricter. Stating the obvious in the face of denial and wishful thinking, Willett and Stampfer noted that "few in the general U.S. population are at an increased risk of death from excessive leanness."

By the time Willett and Stampfer had published their work, however, the "Andres thesis," as it became known, had gathered speed and weight. The notion that excessive leanness was the problem and that overly severe weight guidelines were unfair played to the decade's overwrought identity politics, to concerns about gender, race, ethnicity, and age. In the academy and on the street, people heard what they wanted to hear, and what they wanted to hear was that it was okay to be fatter. And by the time the USDA's Dietary Guidelines Committee met in 1989, what the people wanted to hear had fused with the professional agenda of some of the nation's leading public health scholars.

The personification of that fusion was Dr. C. Wayne Callaway, an esteemed Washington, D.C., physician and public health expert. Callaway had been appointed by the Dietary Guidelines Committee to spearhead an inquiry into weight guidelines. Easygoing, witty, charming, and agile in the logic department, Callaway quickly made his charge a forum for his own inclinations on a wide range of weight-related issues. This was not unusual; most appointees to most public bodies do the same thing, sometimes overtly, sometimes not so. And for the most part, Callaway was on target. It was Callaway who argued for and won one of the most important changes in the guidelines — the inclusion of fat distribution patterns as a key determinate of weight-related risk. As he liked to say, "I can line up ten people, all of the same height and weight, and the fat deposition patterns will be all over the place. What the science shows is that the ones who look more like a pear — who carry their excess weight on their hips — are not as unhealthy as those who look like an apple — the ones who carry the excess fat on their belly." For the first time, Americans were instructed exactly how to calculate their waist-to-hip ratio — an important piece of information when determining whether one should lose weight or not.

But the waist-to-hip ratio also illustrated Callaway's one weakness: a tendency to want to salve too many special constituencies. The ratio was not only medically important, he argued in committee meetings. It was also socially just. Using simplistic weight-for-height tables, he said, "lets men off the hook too easily" (because they carry their excess weight in their belly) while simultaneously discriminating against women (who tend to carry their excess weight in their hips). To make them both use the same table caused women to worry too much and gave men "too much balm." Callaway's understanding of women as a group needing, in some areas, its own health guidelines was sound, but from here his tendency to placate constituencies began to separate him from the data.

There was, for instance, his concern about excessive dieting, a legitimate (albeit epidemiologically small) issue that colored other, more substantive concerns about obesity. In discussing one section about weight control, he interjected, to the surprise of his colleagues, that the committee should leave out the statement "One thing is definite. To lose weight, you must take in fewer calories than you burn." To Callaway, such a statement was "authoritarian." He went on: "What is hidden in that is blaming the victim. There are thousands and thousands of people who are chronically dieting, and if they take in fewer calories, it doesn't help them." At this even his usually sympathetic colleague University of California at Davis nutrition scholar Barbara Schneeman interjected: "But that concept still has to be conveyed to people, that ultimately it *is* caloric balance that will determine weight loss!"

Anorexia and bulimia, also legitimate (and also epidemiologically small) health issues, were also accorded undue emphasis. "Because if we look at certain subsegments of the population," Callaway went on, "as has been done for instance in affluent suburban school systems . . . fourth-grade girls are already dieting and defining themselves as being overweight. So if we come back to this thing about the potential for harm, I think we really need to balance that *and almost give it equal balance.*"

Then came the issue of age. As Callaway saw it, "By the time a woman gets to age sixty-five, only about 10 percent of women are at the quote, ideal body weight." Rather than seeing this as more evidence that Americans were growing fatter, Callaway declared it an issue of inequality. "So, again, we have this age discrimination," he said. "So again, we're using a standard which doesn't make sense to the elderly population." The answer, he said, was to revise the weight guidelines upward — a historic first in the annals of the committee.

But unlike his advocacy of waist-to-hip ratios, Callaway's age-adjusted tables rested on a single — and very shaky — leg: Reubin Andres's 1985 study. Willett and Stampfer tried to get their concerns across, but since they were not members of the committee, "our views did not get a fair shake," Stampfer says.

Willett recalls the situation somewhat more bitterly. "As far as I am concerned," he says, that decision "was one of the worst cases of backroom dealing that I have ever seen." The committee, he says, refused to look at the smoking data, despite the then grow-ing evidence that Andres had been wrong.

Instead, in November of 1990, the committee announced its new guidelines. As the *New York Times* put it, "The guideline on weight suggests that people over thirty-five can be heavier than young adults without risk to health." Andres and Callaway had triumphed. It was okay to get fatter as one aged.

For the next five years, Willett, Stampfer, and a broad swath of the nutrition community labored for better data on the subject of age and weight. Other groups in the United States and abroad, appalled by the committee's action, published new data on the age-weight link as well. Almost all came to similar conclusions: For healthy people, male or female, it is almost always better to avoid weight gain — at any age, for any reason. So convincing was the evidence that, when the committee reconvened in 1995 (sans Callaway), it unanimously voted to rescind the age guide-lines. "Based on published data, there appears to be no justifica-tion for the establishment of a cut point that increases with age," the new committee wrote in a terse note. "Although the nadir of mortality curves increases with age in several studies, these stud-ies have failed to control for a history of smoking, which appears to affect mortality at all ages." Again, it was not okay to gain weight as one got older.

Yet for five years, such was the governmental advice that Americans, experiencing the biggest increases in obesity rates ever, seem very much to have taken to heart. And waist.

Given the debacle of the early 1990s reforms, one would imagine that the American exercise establishment might think twice about proclaiming new public health messages that sanctioned sloth, gluttony, or denial. But about that one would be wrong; they did not think twice. Instead, the brightest lights of their leadership embarked upon another crusade, this one to convince the American public that they should not focus on fat at all — that they should forget about dieting and losing weight and instead learn how to be "fit and fat."

The gladiator of the crusade is Steven Blair, a brilliant Texas epidemiologist, director of the Cooper Institute, and himself a leading proponent of the health-based fitness recommendations of the 1980s. For two decades, Blair has been at the primordial center of the debate about fitness. It has also been something of a personal issue for him. He is, as he likes to say, "Fat, fit, and bald — and none of those things are likely to change."

For years Blair did try to change; in the 1980s he followed a strict diet — the one recommended by the AMA — but to little avail. Like some obese people, his body is in thrall to a stronger genetic inclination to retain excess weight. Unlike most obese people, Blair's response to his birthright has been to get tougher — he is a marathoner, triathlete, and vigorous sportsman. He has run, by his own estimate, more than 80,000 miles over the past thirty years. With his confident, engaging manner, mile-long vita, and persuasive debate style, Blair is his own best advertisement for his fit and fat campaign. And campaign he does. "We've got to get rid of this focus on weight," he likes to say at every media interview. "There's a misdirected focus on weight and weight loss — the focus is all wrong. It's fitness that's the key." Or: "Let's throw away all the scales. Let's stop talking about weight." At times he goes even further, proclaiming that "you can stay overweight and obese if you are fit and be just as healthy, in terms of mortality risk, as a lean fit person."

As usual, the scientific basis for Blair's case rests on studies of clients of the Cooper Institute — white, affluent, male professionals who had come to the center for a medical exam between 1970 and 1989. In Blair's clinical measure of their health, the key variable was fitness as assessed on a treadmill test. The test starts at a speed of eighty-eight meters a minute at zero elevation, which is increased to 2 percent elevation for the second minute, then 1 percent each minute to twenty-five minutes; after that researchers turn up the speed every minute until the test is halted when the subject becomes exhausted. Since total time on a treadmill correlates strongly with individual fitness levels, Blair was then able to assign participants to different, age-group-specific fitness categories — low fit, moderate fit, and high fit. He next calculated in BMI — a weight-for-height index based on health outcomes rather than on "what is normal" — thereby creating three distinct groups to study: normal weight men with low, medium, and high fitness rates; overweight men with low, medium, and high fitness rates; and obese men with low, medium, and high fitness rates.

To find out what all this meant, Blair then figured in the rate of death and related risks that took place within this group over the years. What he found was important. Death rates were inversely related to fitness status. While it wasn't too surprising that high-fit, normal-weight men had death rates 61 percent lower than low-fit men, it was notable that the risk reduction held up when applied to fat men who were in the fit — or high treadmill time — category. The conclusion, in its invariable unexciting academese, was that "inverse gradients of mortality across fitness groups were similar for obese and non-obese men." Blair, however, spun it like this: Fat men who were fit lived longer than slim men who were not fit.

This Blair used to attack U.S. weight guidelines, which he regarded as too restrictive. (The 1995 guidelines suggested that Americans maintain a healthy weight, preferably a BMI of 25 or under.) To sharpen his epidemiological blade, Blair did another study. This time he calculated in risk from cardiovascular disease. The results were again revealing. Fit but overweight men displayed a similar rate of mortality as physically fit men of normal weight. Almost as important, he proclaimed, fit overweight men had a lower risk for cardiovascular disease than unfit normal-weight men. This, of course, was a bit like comparing apples and oranges (or, more apt, apples and bananas); no one, after all, had ever said that being unfit and skinny was a good public health goal. But Blair saw fit to spin it like this: "The health benefits of normal weights appear to be limited to men who have moderate or high levels of cardiorespiratory fitness. These data suggest that the 1995 U.S. weight guidelines may be misleading. . . ." And again: "We do emphasize that increasing fitness may be more important than maintaining healthy weights."

The media translation was predictable. As the Associated Press (and many others) slugged it: "Study finds obese exercisers outlive thin people who don't." A book came out that was entitled *You Don't Have to Be Thin to Win.* The *New York Times* even went so far as to say that Blair had "dispelled" a "myth" that fat people could not be fit.

But that was never really the myth, and that was certainly not why body weight guidelines promoted leanness. Body weight guidelines — and the entire infrastructure of promoting weight loss — lay in long, deep, and convincing science that body weight is inversely related to health. Over and over, studies show: The fatter you are, the more likely you are to be sick, feel sick, and die young. Blair's own data are a case in point. Taking out the fitness variable and looking at body weight only, Blair admitted: "Men with a BMI of >30 were generally less physically fit and had more unfavorable risk factors than men in the lower BMI groups." Lower weight men had higher good cholesterol, lower bad cholesterol, and higher treadmill times than fatter men. "The highest death rate," he added, "was observed among those men in the highest BMI category and correspondingly lower death rates were observed in each subsequently lower BMI category." And when one looks at the *difference* between low fit men in all categories — which one might think would be useful since most obese people are not fit — Blair's upbeat message fades: Normal weight nonfit men had an age-adjusted death rate (the number of excess deaths in the studied group) of 52.1; unfit fat men had the higher rate of 62.1. More: Unfit lean men were half as likely to have a history of hypertension than unfit fat men. In the real world, even according to Blairism, the fat are more likely to die early — and to live precariously — than the lean.

Now look at the fat fit vs. the lean fit in Blair's population. In almost every category, it is better — far better — to be lean. Consider treadmill time. The data are unequivocal: As a person gets fatter, *even if he is getting technically fitter,* he is also less likely to perform as well on the treadmill test as his leaner brothers. Blair admitted: "Men who were normal weight and physically fit had the longest average treadmill time."

But the single most important fact — again detailed by Blair himself — is this: The fat are always less *likely* to be fit than are the lean. The absolute numbers bear this out. Of Blair's total universe of people, 8100 of the lean were fit, 6000 of the overweight were fit, and only 3307 of the obese were fit. But that did not make the editorial — or cultural — cut either. Neither did the fact that those 3307 almost certainly had to work a lot harder to get that fitness. They could likely do that only because they were, as a group, much richer than most Americans. Remember, Blair's real message, almost always lost on its readers, is largely one of class: Yes, you can be fit and fat if you are rich, white, and male. As, again, were all members of the Cooper population.

It would take a hard heart to say it is wrong to tell fat people that they can become fitter by exercising more. They can become fitter. There is also nothing wrong — and everything right — with preaching a doctrine of self-acceptance to go along with that advice. One should not hate oneself because one is fat. But one should not be led to delusion. Weight matters. It always matters. If one is obese, losing weight is key to obtaining optimal health.

There may, however, be something downright cruel about implying that "anyone" can be fit and fat, especially when the principal examples of that are rich white people who have the time, money, and energy to train — not for ten minutes three times a day — but for marathons. Marathons!

Consider a typical example, inevitably trotted out by Blair for some poor general-interest reporter who needs an example of how one can be fit and fat.

His name is David Alexander. Over the past seventeen years he has finished 276 triathlons in 37 countries. He trains so much that he sleeps only four and one half hours a night in order to do so. In a week, Alexander will swim 5 miles, run 30, and cycle 200, and on top of that might compete in not one but two triathlons. Alexander is also, at 5'8" and 260 pounds, "a big boy," he likes to say, "and I'm always going to be big, but I'm healthy." Only much later on in the story do we find out why he is healthy. Alexander is the co-owner of an oil company. There he inhabits an office, we are told, where he sits "surrounded by the antique maps he collects." As is the case of most Americans, for Dave Alexander, fitness is purchased.

But is he really fit? What of the illnesses that derive from fatness that have nothing to do with cardiovascular health? What about type 2 diabetes? On that count the most recent scientific literature is sobering and clear: Alexander is much more likely to get it than he would were he leaner. As a study by Harvard's Departments of Epidemiology and Nutrition and Schools of Public Health concluded in 2001: "The most important risk factor for type 2 diabetes was the body mass index . . . Even a body mass index at the high end of the normal range was associated with a substantially higher risk [than a lower body mass]." How substantial? "More than 61 percent of all cases could be directly attributed to overweight." Although some studies have shown that exercise can somewhat mitigate those risks in fat people, the overwhelming consensus among diabetes experts is perhaps best summed up by a quotation from the director of a New York medical program trying to treat the disease. "Bring me a fat man," this physician told the *Times,* "and I'll show you a diabetic, or someone who will become one."

Excess abdominal fat cells are troublesome in and of themselves for another reason: They are, metabolically, the laboratory of so-called Syndrome X. The syndrome, first identified by the Stanford endocrinologist Gerald Reaven, acts as the precursor to both type 2 and, eventually, full-blown insulin-dependent diabetes. Excess weight is implicated in its progression. This is because, in at least 30 percent of all Americans, insulin-resistant fat cells in the gut produce excess fatty acids, which wreak havoc by attacking the body's vital sugar- and fat-processing functions. The more insulin-resistant fat cells, the more destructive fatty acids. This in turn results in everything from hyperinsulinemia (leading to diabetes) to excess blood fats (leading to artery-clogging) to constricted blood flow (leading to hypertension). Although particularly rampant among the poor and recently modernized peoples of the world (and of those in the United States, as described more fully in chapter 6), the syndrome knows no economic barrier when it comes to fat. Fat cells are its engine, fuelmaker, and distribution network.

As a person ages, excess weight becomes problematic for another reason: bone disease, which it can both cause and complicate. Osteoarthritis of the knee is a case in point. Being heavy drives the progression of this painful disease. A pound of extra body weight places from two to four pounds of extra stress on the knees and hips, even during routine movement, let alone the stress of marathon-like exercise regimes. In the arthritic knee, which takes the majority of the pounding, that stress causes the cartilage to wear away, letting exposed bone surfaces grind against one another. That brings even more swelling, pain, and difficulty in moving about in general.

And that, however the epidemiologists cut it, just ain't fit.

But then, by millennium's end, most Americans were not fit. They were exercising less, eating more — and, thanks to the permissive culture they had created — not feeling very bad about it, thank you very much. It was, after all, a comfortable world, one where a bit of housework sufficed for exercise, where it was okay to gain weight as one aged, where it was healthy to be fat, where the medical consequences of their behavior seemed remote. Even though those consequences were exploding right under their noses.

5

·················

WHAT FAT IS,
WHAT FAT ISN'T

B Y THE MID-1990S the consequences of boundary-less America were everywhere apparent. Physicians in inner-city hospitals were seeing unprecedented numbers of children with type 2 diabetes. (Until then type 2 had been a disease seen almost exclusively in adults.) In the medical literature, obesity was declared a main cause of soaring rates of early puberty among girls as young as nine years old. Fatness also lay behind a disturbing rise in the rate of *Pseudotumor cerebri,* which, as its name denotes, is a brain tumor–like condition, often found in obese women. Weight-induced sleep apnea, hypertension, and arthritis of the knee were on the rise too.

Yet as the studies trickled in, and as various interest groups parsed their meaning, one fact stuck out above all others, at least to those who were on the front lines of studying and treating the phenomenon: In late-twentieth-century America, it was the poor, the underserved, and the underrepresented who were most at risk from excess fat.

While new studies, particularly those from the CDC, showed that the fat epidemic was slowly but surely crossing over into the middle and upper middle classes, particularly among men, the most consistent numbers concerned the poor and the working poor. Among these classes, obesity was rampant. At the very bottom end were households with less than $10,000 of annual income; among them, 33 percent of blacks were obese, 26 percent of Hispanics, and 19 percent of whites. For households with $20,000 to $25,000 in annual income, the rates were substantially lower; 27 percent of blacks, 18 percent of Hispanics, and 20 percent of whites were obese. At the $50,000 and above mark, the rate of blacks who were obese fell to 23 percent, Hispanics rose to 22 percent (perhaps reflecting the prototypical response to new middle-class status), and whites fell to 16 percent.

Culture, ethnicity, gender, and race, of course, also play their roles in determining obesity rates. Black girls and their mothers, for example, tend to be heavier than their white counterparts regardless of income level. Such findings have driven researchers to look deeply for what might be behind such a variable. Was it the long-held (but bogus) notion that blacks are more comfortable being fat? No. Was it, as one scholar proposed, because being fat was a way for a young woman to keep predatory young men at bay? No. The reason, a group of epidemiologists from the University of Pittsburgh concluded, was money. "The relationship of income and obesity [among black girls] . . . appears to be more akin to that of white girls in the 1960s and even to that of traditional societies," they wrote. "What we observe . . . may be a reflection of a differential social development in our society, where a certain lag period may need to elapse between an era when food availability is a concern to an era of affluence with no such concern before an inverse relationship between socioeconomic status and obesity [among blacks] can be seen." In other words, blacks still have not caught up to whites economically, and so still think about food as if scarcity were just around the corner.

The point is not that culture or race does not matter. They do. The point is that class almost always comes first in the equation: class confounded by culture, income inhibited by race or gender, buying power impinged on by ethnicity or immigration status. But why are the numbers of the obese poor suddenly soaring so? One answer is that the same culture that had made possible the huge gains in middle-class obesity is also at work among the poor. Being poor may even magnify the effect. The poor, after all, lead lives that are more episodic than those of the more affluent. They are more likely to experience disruptions in health care, interruptions in income. Food, and the ability to buy it, comes in similar episodes — periods of feeling flush, periods of being on the brink of an empty pantry. The impulse is to eat for today, tomorrow being a tentative proposition at best.

Consider the situation among the poor in the nation's capital. There, obesity has become the defining metropolitan aesthetic. One of D.C.'s most popular clothing stores is Ashley Stewart, a national discount chain specializing in plus-size clothing. Fast food is also ubiquitous — on the street and in the schools. Fast food in the schools, in fact, seems to be a matter of pride. When the D.C. inspector general publicly criticized one school principal for selling fast food on campus, he was immediately shouted down by a number of elected public officials, who defended the principal by saying that he was merely being "enterprising."

The less visible signs of the D.C. obesity epidemic are even more troubling. At Howard University hospital, physicians doing their preliminary patient workups must often use the scale in the downstairs laundry room; it is the only one in the hospital big enough to weigh some of the patients coming in for obesity-related ailments. In the winter of 1999 physicians at the same hospital witnessed something they thought they would never see: a fifteen-year-old girl who died from an enlarged heart. The girl weighed 400 pounds.

There is another factor driving the D.C. poor toward obesity as well, one rarely talked about in public health circles, let alone in the mainstream media. It is what might be called the pain of poverty. As Stephanie Mencimer, a reporter for the *Washington City Paper* who spent several months talking to poor, obese D.C. residents, put it: "The adolescents who started appearing in D.C. hospitals with diabetes four years ago were born almost exactly at the beginning of the last big noninfectious inner-city epidemic. Crack cocaine changed the inner city and its residents in profound ways. Even those poor families that weren't succumbing to the ravages of drug addiction were touched by its side effects: unrelenting violence, the disappearance of vast numbers of men into the criminal justice system, and the emptying out of the neighborhoods." Mencimer cites Dr. Gloria WilderBraithwaite of the Georgetown Mobile Pediatric Clinic: "It's tiresome being poor. Living in the cocoon of obesity is a very comfortable thing to do."

Much of that cocoon has been built especially for the poor by the fast-food industry, which for the past twenty years has emphasized development of the inner-city consumer. As various critics have duly noted in recent years, the push began in the early 1970s, when nascent chains were looking for markets to complement their growing lock on suburban customers. Fortunately for the companies, the federal government — through the newly created Small Business Administration (SBA) — had gone into the loan-making business, with a special emphasis on urban redevelopment. In particular, the agency wanted to empower minority entrepreneurs by guaranteeing loans for new businesses. The consequent gold rush went beyond anyone's wildest expectations. By 1979 the SBA had guaranteed eighteen thousand franchise loans, with fast-food outlets a leading beneficiary. Many of those franchises flopped, with the American taxpayer left to eat the remaining unpaid loans, but many of these new outlets thrived. That drove the policy forward, even through twelve years of Reagan and Bush, both of whom ran ostensibly anti-SBA administrations. In 1996, according to a study by the conservative Heritage Foundation, the policy was still in high gear. That year the SBA guaranteed almost $1 billion in new franchise loans, with more — six hundred — going to the fast-food segment than any other. No wonder that, by the late 1990s, one in four fast-food burgers was purchased by a consumer in the inner city.

That many of these new consumers were teenagers was no chance phenomenon. McDonald's had already laid the groundwork for their allegiance in the mid-1970s, when it introduced the Happy Meal. The concept was pioneered by a little-known Kansas City ad executive named Bob Bernstein, who had noticed that parents increasingly were bringing their children along with them to McDonald's — and then sharing their own meals instead of buying one for Junior. That, Bernstein recalls, presented both a problem and an opportunity. "We knew that kids would want — demand — their own meals if one was available." Bernstein then got an idea for what would eventually become the Happy Meal formula — "putting at least ten things on the bag that a kid could read" — from his own child, whom he observed reading the cereal box every morning. "It was very simple. I asked him why he read the box, and he said, 'Dad, it's just something to do while I eat breakfast.'" As any contemporary parent knows, the Happy Meal became one of the company's most enduring (if annoying) success stories.

But for McDonald's it was not enough simply to cue young children when they were small and then rely on adult advertising to keep them as loyal customers later on. By the mid-1980s, with the value meal concept at competing fast-food chains chipping away at the core McDonald's audience, the company decided it needed a new strategy to capture and retain "tweens," or pre-teens. This it did by forcing its advertising agencies to come up with new ways to measure the impact of youth advertising. The effort was so important that, in March 1986, the company sent its head media buyer, Karen Dixon-Ware, to reprimand the entire Media Research Club of Chicago. Bad Nielsen and Arbitron numbers on children would no longer be tolerated, Dixon-Ware told the stunned audience. Attributing fluctuations in children's viewing habits to "simply the fickleness of children," she lectured, "is a cop-out." The agencies had better find a way to get "tween" viewers' attention or risk losing the McDonald's account.

The reaction to the speech was immediate and industry-wide.

Arbitron and Nielsen rating systems and the viewer diaries they are based upon were retooled to better capture demographic data on children's viewing patterns. The new data convinced McDonald's and its imitators to allocate more money for tween-centric ads. Soon there was so much money for youth advertising that entire new ad agencies were formed simply to handle the "Saturday A.M. buy." Corporate identities were remade, or "tweened." Pizza Hut changed its longtime jingle "Pizza Hut and nothing more" to "More rock 'n' roll, more fun." As its marketing director, Humphrey Kadaner, explained to *Advertising Age,* the change was "targeted specifically to kids." Attracting a host of other junk-food purveyors, such ads eventually became the dominant background noise of all morning programming for children. As a team of Columbia University researchers reported, by 1993, 41 percent of all Saturday morning kid show ads were for high-fat foods. What was once a time for children to get a few laughs on a non–school day had become a time to indoctrinate them on the benefits of grease, salt, and ever increasing amounts of sugar. About this the Federal Trade Commission and the Federal Communications Commission, the two regulatory agencies that might have buffered the tween revolution, said nothing and did nothing.

One reason for that inactivity — or at least one often cited as a justification for inaction — was a lack of hard, empirical data about fast-food consumption and its relationship to increased energy intake. In other words, does using fast-food restaurants frequently result in a child — or anyone — consuming more calories over time? On this issue the obesity establishment, the nexus of advocacy, scientific, and policy organizations focused on the issue, has been strangely quiet. Or quiescent. In its leading journals of the past decade one can count on two hands the number of articles studying fast food. Part of the reason is pragmatic; with limited funds and endless battles to fight, groups like the North American Association for the Study of Obesity (NAASO) and the International Association for the Study of Obesity (IASO) see a fight with McDonald's as ultimately unproductive.

("What, are we going to convince them to stop selling french fries?" one member told me at a recent NAASO convention.) There is also a kind of institutional pragmatism at work; many makers of candy, soft drinks, and other less than desirable products often support the promotion of health and fitness.

But in 2001 a group of epidemiologists from the University of Minnesota broke with conventional wisdom and published an in-depth report on the association between fast-food use and caloric intake. Studying almost 5000 adolescent students in thirty-one urban secondary schools, the researchers tracked their use of fast-food restaurants through daily dietary diaries. The results were striking. A boy who never ate at a fast-food restaurant during the school week averaged a daily calorie count of 1952; one who ate fast food one to two times a week (as did more than half of all the children in the study) consumed an average of 2192 calories a day; while those who ate fast food three times or more a week (one fifth of the studied) consumed an amazing 2752 calories a day. "Fast food restaurant use was positively associated with intake of total energy, percent energy from fat, daily servings of soft drinks . . . and was inversely associated with daily servings of fruit, vegetables, and milk," the researchers concluded. Worse, they added, "eating habits established in adolescence, including preference for and reliance on fast food, may place them at future risk for higher fat and energy intake as they move into young adulthood, a developmental period that is high risk for increased sedentary behaviors and excess weight gain."

By the mid-1990s another grim example of obesity among the poor appeared in Appalachia, traditionally ground zero in the war against *under*nutrition in America. There, studying elementary school children in a low-income township in eastern Kentucky, the anthropologist Deborah Crooks was astonished to find stunting and obesity not just present but prevalent. Among her subjects, 13 percent of girls were stunted — they were shorter than 95 percent of all other U.S. children in their age group; 33 percent of all children were significantly overweight; and 13 percent of the children were obese — 21 percent of the boys and 9 percent of the girls.

A sensitive, elegant writer who had originally been attracted to the study of nutrition through an interest in impoverished Third World populations, Crooks drew from her work three important conclusions: One, that poor children in the United States often face the same evolutionary nutritional pressures as those in newly industrializing nations, where traditional diets are displaced by high-fat diets and where, as in the United States, laborsaving technology reduces physical activity. Second, Crooks found that "height and weight are cumulative measures of growth . . . reflecting a sum total of environmental experience over time." Last, and perhaps most important, Crooks concluded that while stunting might be partly explained by individual household conditions — income, illness, education, and marital status — obesity "may be more of a community-related phenomenon." A town's physical and economic infrastructures — safe playgrounds, access to high-quality, low-cost food, and transportation to recreation facilities — were the real determinants of physical activity levels, and, hence, weight. "Given that as a nation, we are trying to improve public health by promoting more healthful behaviors," she concluded, "this research indicates that nutrition education efforts might benefit from a greater focus on children. . . . These efforts should also address the particular concerns of communities and families in poverty."

Poverty. Class. Income. Over and over, these emerged as the key determinants of obesity and weight-related disease. True, there was a new trend that saw significant numbers of the middle and upper middle class also experiencing huge weight gains. But the basic numbers were — and are — clear and consistent; the largest concentrations of the obese, regardless of race, ethnicity, and gender, reside in the poorest sectors of the nation — among the chronically impoverished (from Appalachia to the rural South), among the working poor (from L.A. barrios to New York's Little

Puerto Rico), and among what might be called the structurally poor (from Detroit's housing projects to reservation-tied Native Americans). Here is the definitive *Handbook on Obesity:* "In heterogeneous and affluent societies like the United States, there is a strong inverse correlation of social class and obesity." From the *Annals of Epidemiology:* "In white girls . . . both TV viewing and obesity were strongly inversely associated with household income as well as with parental education." And, again, from the *Handbook,* this time from the leading international epidemiologists on the subject: "The increase in the prevalence of obesity occurred in all income groups but was relatively largest in the poorest groups. In 1974 the women with the highest income were heaviest whereas in 1989 the women with the middle income were the heaviest. There were strong positive correlations [with obesity] between family income in the poorest and middle-income families."

Yet in America of the 1990s class seemed to be the last thing on the minds of most public intellectuals dealing with obesity. Instead, the tendency of many in the academy was to fetishize or "postmodernize" the problem. To trivialize it. A good example — and a bad diet — can be found in Richard Klein's 1996 *Eat Fat.* In it, Klein, a professor of French at Cornell University who has struggled with weight gain for most of his life, proposed that people simply stop trying to avoid fat and instead, as his title suggests, indulge in it with wild abandon. "Believe me, it isn't easy — today, in our culture, with all the messages coming down to eat no fat, less fat, low or lite fat, [or] to eat fat free," Klein writes. "But this is a postmodern diet book. What it's proposing is something like an anti-diet. Try this for six weeks: EAT FAT."

Then, after 242 pages of postmodern navel-gazing, Klein, confronted with a modern reality, is forced to completely reverse his own prescription. In a hastily written postscript he confesses: "With the sort of irony that reinforces my belief in the unconscious, as I was writing this book, I was confronted in my personal life with a drama surrounding fat, which contradicts my book's conclusions. My mother had become so fat that it pressed on her lungs while she slept . . . fat was her greatest enemy. How could I tell my mother to EAT FAT? I had to admit that under these circumstances, the most responsible thing I could do as a son was to say to my mother, EAT RICE." Ms. Klein promptly lost twenty pounds, and her once life-threatening case of sleep apnea abated.

Yet Klein's postmodern musings — and the fact that they were so fondly received by the tittering masses in the humanities — are a perfect reflection of how the media of the 1990s tended to interpret obesity — namely, as everything *but* a class and medical issue.

Consider the reaction to a 1995 study by a group of University of Arizona researchers, published in the journal *Human Organization*. Looking for evidence that black girls and white girls viewed their bodies in "dramatically different ways," the group documented that while 90 percent of white junior high and high school girls voiced "some dissatisfaction" with their weight, a full 70 percent of African American girls were "satisfied" with their bodies. Although one reading of this might reasonably be that black girls had come uncritically to accept — and even celebrate — a condition that would one day almost certainly lead to a variety of serious medical problems, the mainstream press, almost without exception, chose a different angle: to celebrate the "good news." As *Newsweek* proclaimed, "After decades of preaching black is beautiful, black parents and educators have gotten across the message of self-respect. Indeed, black teens grow up equating a full figure with health and fertility." *Newsweek*'s journalist, Michelle Ingrassia, was so happy about this that she went out to find a fifteen-year-old black male from Harlem to co-sign the celebration. "You got be real fat for me to notice," the young man said. This, Ingrassia concluded, was because other new studies had indicated something even more celebratory — that "black men send some of the strongest signals for black girls to be fat."

For years, the "black men want big women and black girls feel good about being fat" doctrine dominated most popular discussion of fatness in the African American community. Often, it had the effect of pre-empting serious discussion of obesity's medical impact on black Americans. Instead, obese black girls became a vehicle for doing something that the media was increasingly happy to do: bash slim culture. (As one network affiliate commentator I watched one evening proclaimed, "Here is one group of girls who couldn't care less about looking like Kate Moss!") Uncritical acceptance of the doctrine even led some to propose a separate system for treating the black obese. Writing in the *Journal of the American Dietetic Association,* the authors Melnyk and Weinstein, after endless hand-wringing, eventually worked themselves up enough to admit the need for early intervention in cases of adolescent obesity. But only, they insisted, if the approach were grounded in "black belief systems." The priority, they wrote, should be "to eliminate a predominantly white Anglo Saxon ethnocentric viewpoint to prevent and treat obesity."

Beyond the twisted uses of the African American fatness doctrine, just how true were the data behind it? For the past five years social scientists studying the question have come away with one answer: not very. In 1999 a reassessment of the key early data that the doctrine was based upon was presented in the journal *Perceptual and Motor Skills.* The authors wanted to find out if the respondents to the original study had been overinfluenced by their own body weight; were the so-called "racial differences" in self-perception and other-perception really just differences in how fat people see the world versus how normal or thin people view the world, regardless of race? After adjusting for respondents' weight, the data could corroborate only *one* of the original studies' nineteen supposed differences between African and European American females (the importance of silky hair for European Americans). And one of the most celebrated "differences" between black girls and white girls dissolved entirely. "The importance of round buttocks for African American women disappeared when controlling for respondents' weight," the authors concluded.

There was more. It was true that, in the initial study, African American men preferred larger body types in their African American mates than did Anglo males. But that difference — of about ten pounds — was manifest within an overall desired "universe" not of fatness, but of thinness. In other words, both black men and white men preferred thin women; it was merely their definition of what constituted thin that differed. As the researchers found, "Men and women, regardless of race, prefer slightly thin and average body types." Other age groups were restudied as well, and, again, when it came to the notion that black Americans were "comfortable" with being fat, the data cut the other way. In the year 2000, looking at 1086 male and female college students of all races at California State University at Los Angeles, psychologists at that school showed that "although it has been proposed that certain subcultures show greater acceptance of overweight and less tolerance of thinness and underweight in women, our findings demonstrate no significant race differences between women or men in different ethnic groups."

Does all of this matter? Increasingly, those who study the subject of self-perception and obesity argue that it does. A report in the journal *Clinical Pediatrics* looked at the self-images of an indigent, predominantly black population of children and the relationship of those self-images to their weight. The results were revealing. Thirty-nine percent of the girls and 67 percent of the boys were significantly overweight. Females tended to view themselves as fatter and males perceived themselves as thinner than their actual composition. Parents were "highly inaccurate" in perceiving such overweight, particularly when it came to their sons. The kids themselves "did not recognize the importance of exercise." This was hardly something to celebrate as a victory for black pride, leading the authors to conclude, in uncharacteristically blunt terms, that "bodyfat measurement and counseling *should be done at an early age to improve this remarkable lack of perception about obesity*" (emphasis added).

The common response to such recommendations often boils down to: Won't that make black girls just as weight-obsessed as white girls? "That's the big conundrum," says Richard MacKenzie, a physician who treats overweight and obese girls at Children's Hospital in downtown L.A. "No one wants to overemphasize the problems of being fat to these girls, for fear of creating body image problems that might lead to anorexia and bulimia." Speaking anecdotally, he adds: "The problem with that is this: For every one affluent white anorexic you create by 'overemphasizing' obesity, you foster ten obese poor girls by downplaying the severity of the issue." Judith Stern, a professor of nutrition and internal medicine at the University of California at Davis, is more blunt about this issue. "The number of kids with eating disorders is positively dwarfed by the numbers with obesity. It sidesteps the whole class issue. We've got to stop that and get on with the real problem."

Moreover, such sidestepping denies poor minority girls a principal — if sometimes unpleasant — psychological incentive to lose weight: that of social stigma. Only recently has the academy come to grapple with this. Writing in a recent issue of the *International Journal of Obesity,* the scholar S. Averett looked at the hard numbers: 44 percent of African American women weigh more than 120 percent of their recommended body weight, yet are less likely than whites to perceive themselves as overweight. Anglo women, poor and otherwise, registered higher anxiety about fatness, and experienced far fewer cases of chronic obesity. "Social stigma may serve to control obesity among white women," Averett reluctantly concluded. "If so, the physical and emotional effects of greater pressure to be thin must be weighed against reduced health risks associated with overweight and obesity."

In other words, perhaps boundaries, an unpleasant but good thing for affluent white people, are also a good thing for poor and middle-class black people.

Even when an occasional healthy thin role model for the poor gets trotted out, the modern media are apt to use her not as a goad to trim down, but as a justification to stay fat. Consider the lengthy cultural discussion that took place in 1999 over the "meaning" of actress Jennifer Lopez's ample derriere. The debate began when *Vanity Fair* published a photo, taken from behind, of the actress wearing nothing but tight, lace-up underwear. Because Lopez, to paraphrase Raymond Chandler, has a body that "would make a bishop kick a hole in a stained glass window," many sat up and took notice. The *New York Observer* proclaimed, "Ms. Lopez has a nice big muscled butt — a-hoo-ga!"

Immediately a number of large-size ethnic celebrities jumped on the bandwagon to say how great it was that "someone who isn't perfect" was being considered so attractive. So did a number of columnists. Writing in Salon.com, the normally low-key writer Erin Aubry was moved to the literary equivalent of a civil rights march: "Being a black woman with a similar (all right, bigger) endowment, I felt an odd mixture of pride and panic. Was this a passing Hollywood fancy or a giant step for butt-kind? . . . Would my own butt, which I have alternately embraced and lamented and written about extensively as a metaphor for tortuously unrealized black assimilation in America, finally get its aesthetic props?" On *Oprah,* Lopez paraded about in her tight cigarette pants as Oprah checked out Lopez's derriere and proclaimed, "You go, girl, in them pants!"

Yet nowhere did anyone comment on one other reason Jennifer Lopez might be so popular, particularly among young Latinas. Could it simply be that they want to look like her — a perfectly fit, tight-bodied woman, lean from years of professional dancing, with, when all is said and done, a nice but not very big rear end at all? That wouldn't, of course, be "the right way" to see it. But it might be the accurate way.

Gender is the media's other preoccupation when it comes to interpreting obesity. Its origin lies in the tremendous popularity of the 1978 bestseller *Fat Is a Feminist Issue,* which tutored a whole generation of young professionals on the subject. In that book, the British psychotherapist Susie Orbach presented a nuanced, passionate look at female compulsive eating and its roots in patriarchal culture. "Compulsive eating in women is a response to their social position," she wrote. The opposite was also "true": Anorexia, Orbach (and several others) held, derives from modern culture's obsession with unattainable thinness, often in the form of thin models, thin celebrities, and even thin clothing. "Fat is a social disease, and fat is a feminist issue," Orbach wrote. "Fat is not about self-control or lack of will power. . . . It is a response to the inequality of the sexes."

Modern epidemiology to the contrary aside, how true is the underlying notion here — that too much fat awareness somehow causes eating disorders? Once again, the data — and the experience of physicians, health workers, and others in the field — consistently indicate otherwise. The resident historian at Cornell University's Department of Human Development and Family Studies, Joan Jacobs Brumberg, who has written the only thorough, objective history of anorexia, put it this way: "An early and distinctive psychopathology of middle class life, the disease itself [anorexia] preceded the familiar body image imperatives usually associated with it. A historical perspective shows that anorexia nervosa existed before there was a mass cultural preoccupation with dieting and a slim female body."

Not only was anorexia not the fault of the mass media, Brumberg wrote, it was — and is — hardly the "widespread disease" so often proclaimed by its main interest group, the American Anorexia and Bulimia Association (AABA). "The association's materials routinely state that anorexia and bulimia strike a million Americans every year and that 150,000 die annually," Brumberg wrote. But after looking deeply at the epidemiological data, Brumberg arrived at a very different — and more accurate — number, 1.6 per 100,000. So why all the attention? The answer, she wrote, is that most anorexics come from the upper middle class — in her words "a highly specific social address." And that, she concluded, "reflects a basic medical reality — that there are fashions in diagnosis."

There was another thing wrong with the skewed attention to

anorexia, Brumberg wrote. "I am disquieted by the tendency to equate all female mental disorders with political protest. Certainly we need to acknowledge the relationship between sex-role constraints and problematic behaviors in women, but the madhouse is a somewhat troubling site for a female pantheon. To put it another way: as a feminist, I believe that the anorectic deserves our sympathy but not necessarily our veneration."

Yet although no serious scholar has ever challenged Brumberg's numbers, or her class analysis, venerate is exactly what a whole new generation of journalists have chosen to do when it comes to anorexia. Writing in a May 1999 issue of the *New York Times Magazine,* the author Jennifer Egan actually took to comparing the anorectic and the suffering of the modern anorectic to that of Saint Catherine of Siena. Egan's principal example: Princess Di, who, because of her own well-known bouts of anorexia, "can legitimately be called a popular saint." That Egan's saint came from a rather supremely specific social address didn't seem to affect her beatification either.

One reflection of such conflicted notions about obesity can be found in the still strong resistance, in some quarters of the nation, toward body composition tests of school-age children. The tests are usually performed by PE or health education teachers using a small pair of calipers applied to either the calf or triceps muscle. Simple, quick, and relatively unintrusive, the calipers test is one of the few ways a contemporary parent can get objective information about fatness and their child. Yet whenever such programs are initiated, usually by some active, passionate health education teacher, "parents sort of freak out," says Professor J. R. Whitehead, of the Department of Physical Education and Exercise Science at the University of North Dakota. Whitehead, who has studied body composition testing for more than twenty years, acknowledges that part of that reaction is normal — parents don't want anyone touching their child who doesn't absolutely have to touch their child. But some of the reaction is irrational, he says, "like the notion that a fat test will somehow make a kid feel bad about himself and then launch into a lifelong course of anorexia."

To find out if such fears had any basis, Whitehead studied groups of seventh graders. He divided them into three groups. One group received the body composition test and were then taught about the health and medical reasons for such a test; a second group was merely measured; a third, unmeasured, group served as a control. The students then completed a series of scientifically vetted questionnaires, designed to plumb what impact the testing might have had on their self-image or self-esteem. The results were clear. There were no effects "on social physique anxiety," Whitehead concluded. "The results support the premise that skinfold calipers can be used in an educational context to facilitate cognitive learning without causing adverse affective consequences" — without causing bad body images. Similar studies of fifth and sixth graders, and another of college students, came out the same. "I don't come to that conclusion lightly," Whitehead says. "I am as concerned about body image issues as the next parent — I worry about it as regards my own daughter and her friends, but that is not what anyone should fear when it comes to body testing. They should see it as a way to teach kids about one health-fitness measure, and as a possible medical issue."

Another consequence of the obsession about anorexia is to skew the medical system in its favor, and to bias it against treatment and prevention of obesity. Today, there are several safe, effective drugs in the anti-anorexia arsenal. Insurance companies and HMOs recognize their importance, and pay for them as part of a patient's course of treatment. Such is not the case when it comes to obesity. Neither of the approved anti-obesity drugs — Orlistat and Meridia — is considered particularly effective. Neither can be prescribed to children or adolescents. And insurance companies are notoriously resistant to paying for them.

The notion of an obesity drug for children may frighten some, particularly those who remember the poorly administered diet drugs of the past, not to mention the debacle of fen-phen in more recent years. Yet those on the leading edge of obesity treatment believe a drug is essential. "I am convinced that the drug for treating a truly obese child, which we see more and more and more of, will be a lifelong drug," says Francine Kaufman, the new president of the American Diabetes Association, who specializes in such cases. "But we aren't seeing that coming down the tube anytime soon."

In the tube instead are simply more drugs to treat the consequences of obesity, mainly diabetes. Whole companies have been retooled to do so. Such was the case in 1999, when Eli Lilly and Company built its new manufacturing plant. The plant is the largest factory dedicated to the production of a single drug in industry history. The drug is insulin, the sales of which are growing, at least at Lilly, at 24 percent a year.

No wonder, then, that almost every leading pharmaceutical conglomerate has like-minded ventures under way. Many have a special emphasis on pill-form treatments for non–insulin-dependent forms of diabetes. A recent advertisement for the drug Avandia sums up the industry attitude. Showing a photograph of an attractive elderly black man and his son, the ad proclaims, "The 20th century brought him type 2 diabetes . . . the 21st century gave him insulin-sensitizing Avandia." In fact, the market segment is considered so important that any large company executive without a "diabetes portfolio" is considered hopelessly out of touch. As James Kappel, one of Lilly's public relations executives, explains, "These days, you've got to be in diabetes."

Diabetes — the growth industry for an ever expanding nation.

6

·····················

WHAT THE EXTRA
CALORIES DO TO YOU

A T ABOUT THE TIME that traditional inner-city populations and many suburbanites came under the sway of
cheap fast foods, another demographic boon appeared on
the horizon for its most aggressive purveyors. The Latino immigration surge of the mid-1980s was coming of economic age; in
many large cities, from Los Angeles to New York to Chicago,
they were displacing older urban populations and bringing with
them new consumer demands. Almost immediately, every major
fast-food company started a Spanish-language campaign. Once
relegated to the "alternative buy" category, the "Spanish buy"
now became a mainstream buy, with tens of millions of dollars in
new ad budgets designated specifically to capture the Latin consumer.

In Los Angeles, the new Ellis Island, such efforts often became news stories in themselves. In the fall of 1999, on the same
day that the Spanish-language *La Opinión* ran a banner story
headlined DIABETES, EPIDEMIA EN LATINOS, Krispy Kreme
doughnuts opened its newest store in Van Nuys, in the heart of
the San Fernando Valley's burgeoning Latino population. It was,
as they like to say in marketing circles, a "resonant" event, re-

plete with around-the-block lines, celebrity news anchors, and stern cops directing traffic between freebie dunks. Everywhere the Latin flavor was pushed: "Chocolate iced custard filled" became *"Rellena de crema pastelera y cubierta con chocolate."* "Cinnamon apple filled" became *"Rellena de manzana y canela."* With norteño music blaring, the store itself seemed to pulse with excitement.

Yet one corner of the affair seemed a decidedly placid world apart. There sat a young Anglo fellow, eyes red from overwork. It was the new store's manager and marketing director. After a few rather uninspired answers to a reporter's questions, he fielded one about strategy: Why did Krispy Kreme, with all of the pent-up demand for its profitable franchises elsewhere, decide to locate here?

"See," he said, checking his watch and brushing a crumb of choco-glaze from his fingers, "the idea is simple: accessible but not convenient."

"Accessible but not convenient?"

"Eh, yuh," he explained. "See, the idea is to make the store accessible — easy to get into and out of from the street — but just a tad away from the, eh, *mainstream* so as to make sure customers are pre-sold — and very in*tent* — before they get here. We want them in*tent* to get at least a dozen before they even *think* of coming in."

But why this slightly non-"mainstream" place?

"Because it's *obvious* . . ." He gestured to the dozens of stout doughnut enthusiasts queuing around the building. "We're looking for all the bigger families."

Bigger in size?

"Yeah." His eyes rolled, like little glazed crullers. "Bigger in *size*."

Bigger in *size* — but why? After all, if there was ever a population of hardworking, energy-expending people in the United States, it was L.A.'s Latinos. Most of them had come from hardscrabble towns in north and central Mexico and beyond to lead more comfortable — but often just as labor-intensive — lives in the City of Angels. In fact, their hard labor — and the fact that they were un-unionized — was the one thing that made them extra valuable in the constantly changing L.A. labor pool. There their services enabled the middle and upper middle classes to continue their upward, double-income ascent. Latino maids cleaned the house, Latino nannies watched the kids after school, Latino gardeners mowed the lawn and blew the leaves away. Yet if they were expending so much energy, why were they gaining so much weight? The question is a road map to an even bigger concern: How does boundary-free culture, class, free market entrepreneurism, and biology make modern man fat?

One answer might be found in what has become known as the thrifty gene theory, the notion that we, as a species, are genetically programmed to hold on to fat. The theory, first articulated by V. Neel in 1962, argues that the gene most likely implicated is the one that pushes glycogen into muscle tissue; a defect in that gene, or in another one close by, causes that glycogen instead to be stored as fat. It is also known as the insulin-resistance gene. As elegantly restated by Leif Groop, the current leading proponent of the theory, "The insulin-resistance gene has protected individuals during long periods of starving by storing energy as fat rather than as glycogen in muscle. The abundance of food in Western society has made this once protective gene a deleterious one, suggesting that these individuals are not equipped with the metabolic machinery to handle overeating."

Perhaps more important is the way that the thrifty gene expresses itself through and combines with different environmental experiences. The nutritionally poor environment of many men and women born in Mexico and Central America, for example, might accentuate the effects of the thrifty gene and its relatives. One way it might do so is through what scientists now call in utero programming. The theory holds that a pregnant woman who experiences starvation during pregnancy is more likely to have a child that is metabolically disposed to retain fat. Two mechanisms incline that child to do so. One is impaired fat oxidation through alterations in the gene responsible for burning fat. The result: Dietary fat gets stored rather than burned, leading to obesity in later life. The other mechanism is impaired sugar metabolism, which some scientists believe derives from an inadequately developed pancreas in the offspring of starved mothers. The consequence: not enough insulin, with excess sugars either running amok in the bloodstream or being stored as fat.

Barry Bogin, an anthropologist at the University of Michigan at Dearborn, has been watching this process unfold in two groups of Mayan immigrants from Guatemala, one in Indiantown, Florida, the other in Los Angeles, California. "What we are seeing is a mismatch between culture and metabolism," Bogin says. "We are seeing the greatest one-generation gains in height ever — but we are also seeing huge weight gain. Not because of heredity in the classic sense — genetics — but rather because of their metabolic inheritance." As Bogin sees it, that metabolic inheritance derives from a long history of cultural and political oppression, one initiated by European conquerors and now continued by their twenty-first-century descendants in urban Guatemala. Such cultural dominance has reinforced further economic exploitation of the Maya, leading to poverty and then generation after generation of children born to nutritionally deprived mothers. Those children are born with a metabolic inclination to hold on to fat, "which works fine as long as they are in a culture of scarcity," Bogin says. "But in a culture of abundance, it doesn't." Instead, they blow up. "In a strange way, you are seeing the original traumas of conquest being played out, metabolically, in the streets of Los Angeles."

Bogin also notes that the experience of the L.A. Guatemalans fits into what is known about the growth patterns of poor peoples who move to richer nations. Increase in height from generation to generation, he writes, "lags behind increases in weight and body composition. This happens because . . . height reflects health and nutritional history, whereas weight and body composition reflect recent events. Indeed, a child's height is a historical record of both the individual and his or her parents."

Immigrants may also suffer from what might be called the "shantytown syndrome." Studying fifty-eight pre-pubertal boys in a São Paolo, Brazil, slum, epidemiologists from Tufts University were able to document a slightly different source of impaired fat oxidation: childhood undernutrition. Although still somewhat speculative, the state-of-the-art explanation runs thus: Long-term undernutrition is usually accompanied by a reduction in insulin growth factor, or IGF-1. IGF-1 plays an important role in stimulating hormones that accelerate fat oxidation. Therefore, any reduction in concentrations of IGF-1 may also result in decreased fat oxidation. Many first-generation immigrants from Mexico and Central America experienced just such childhood undernutrition, and therefore carry the consequential oxidation impairment to the more nutritionally dense environment of the modern American city. No IGF-1 plus lots of fast food means more obese kids in places like the City of Angels.

Once here, and once fat — Krispy Kreme right in the neighborhood — the immigrant parent is much more likely to produce fat toddlers, another predictor of both childhood and adult obesity. Looking at nineteen studies of birth weight and its relationship to obesity, the British Institute of Children's Health found that "the child of obese parents is at increased risk of becoming fat early in life, and once relatively fat, he/she is more likely to be so later in adulthood." The current obesity rate for Mexican American children would seem to be testimony to that finding. Between the ages of five and eleven, 27.4 percent of Mexican American girls are obese, as are 23 percent of boys. By fourth grade the rate for girls peaks at 32.4 percent. By fifth grade boys top out at 43.4 percent.

Such, then, is one biomedical reaction to the New World, *rellena de crema* style.

*   *   *

If a court case were ever brought to adjudicate the effects of obesity on the human body, the proverbial people's number one would come straight out of the coat pocket of Dr. Scott Loren-Selco, a neurologist at L.A.'s frenetic USC Medical Center, one of the busiest urban hospitals in the nation. Loren-Selco's pocket contains a BMI card. BMI, or body mass index, is a more sophisticated method for determining healthy weight for height, in essence dividing body weight in kilograms by height in meters squared (for a simplified method, see Appendix). Loren-Selco's card thus allows him to easily calculate whether a patient is normal weight, overweight, or obese. "And it's one of the first things I get my patients and their parents familiar with," he says. That's because an increasing number of his young patients are not only obese, but, because of it, have a disease once thought to be solely the woe of adults: type 2 diabetes.

"We are seeing it all the time now, and believe me, it is frightening," he says. "I mean, I tell them all the time that I could take them up to the diabetes ward and show them their possible future: the blind, the amputees, the endless number of people who are completely infirm because of type 2 — and who are all obese."

Loren-Selco understands why he sees more obese youth these days. "The message they are getting, especially in the immigrant population, is what they hear and see via TV — they immediately understand that this is a place about 'more,' where they can get more. It's 'Look at me! I'm just a poor kid from Xapotecas and even I can get more.' They can afford supersized burgers and fries — and so they get them. There's no one out there telling them it is wrong — certainly not the fast-food companies, and, frankly, certainly not most physicians, who still aren't trained in nutrition."

Across town, up in the endocrinology department of Children's Hospital, Dr. Francine Kaufman is also getting — and giving — the proverbial wake-up call. Children had been coming in fat and sick since the early 1990s. "As endocrinologists, all of us were aware of the changing trends, and all of us were somewhat involved in obesity. It was just another part of the job," she explains. "It wasn't even something a lot of us wanted to deal with, because the disease links were not as strong."

That began to change in the mid-1990s, when Kaufman began seeing children like Jason (not his real name). A typical referral from county social services, the fourteen-year-old was poor, unkempt, lacking in the most basic forms of medical care, and slipping into a morass of profound health problems. One other thing: Jason weighed three hundred pounds. He had arrived at Kaufman's office with a note from his school nurse. The nurse directed Kaufman to Jason's "obviously poor" bathing habits. There were, after all, several "dirty" dark patches on the back of his neck, on his elbows, and on his knees — anywhere "dirt" might accumulate. But almost immediately Kaufman could see that Jason was not unclean at all — or at least no more dirty than the average child. The smooth, velvety dark shadings in his skin-fold areas were *Acanthosis nigricans,* a rare skin disease that resulted from too much insulin in the blood. In the past, the disease has been manifest almost entirely in adult populations with diabetes and other severe metabolic disorders. Seeing it on Jason, "we could see that he had never been screened for diabetes, never been adequately evaluated, and here was the school nurse, telling him he had to bathe better." Here, at last, was the classic marker — a link connecting obesity, youth, and diabetes.

By 1996, in pediatric clinics, children's wards, private practices, and teaching universities around the country, physicians were coming to a sobering new conclusion: Type 2 diabetes, a potentially crippling, lifelong chronic disease, had come home to roost among the poor, the young, and the fat. The rate of increase had been swift. In 1992, for example, most pediatric diabetes centers in the United States reported only 2 to 4 percent of their diabetes patients as type 2. Two years later that figure jumped to 16 percent of new cases. By 1999 the figure in some parts of the country would zoom to nearly 45 percent of new cases. Most of the new cases were found in African American, Mexican

American, and Native American youth. Just up the coast from Kaufman, in the coastal town of Ventura, 31 percent of new onset diabetes cases in children were Hispanic. As Kaufman saw it, "Something had changed."

But what? The short answer is that more kids were fat, more kids were fatter, and so more kids were developing conditions caused by excess fat. But to truly understand what had changed, one first has to understand a little about the biology of the obese body.

At the most fundamental level, the obese body is like a four-cylinder car pulling a trailer full of bricks; it is, in the simplest sense, overloaded. Its "cylinders" — the heart and its ancillary arteries and veins — are not built for pulling the extra weight, and so must work harder, straining to accommodate the load. Its fuel injection system — the pancreas, the liver, and all of the organs that process fuel — are similarly overloaded, unable to process enough energy or to get it to the proper place to be used to fire the body's key muscles. Its chassis — the skeleton — groans under the excess weight, and like a car with bad shocks, begins to jangle and bump with the most minute movements.

There, however, ends the car simile, for when it comes to diabetes, there is no mechanical analogue to the human pancreas, the central player in the drama of the disease. A small, elongated organ tucked into the abdomen, the pancreas is responsible for making insulin, and it is insulin that makes sure that nutrients get into muscle cells. In a nondiabetic body, insulin is produced in a region of the pancreas known as the islets of Langerhans, named for the late-nineteenth-century German pathologist who discovered their function. There, "beta" cells secrete the hormone into the bloodstream. Once in the bloodstream, insulin binds to receptors on the surface of tissue cells, in a sense "pushing" those little buttons like doorbells to open the cell door to nutrients in the form of glucose. (Glucose is dietary carbohydrate — sugars — resynthesized by the liver to be used by cells for fuel, or to be stored as glycogen for later use.) The cell then "burns" the fuel, using it to repair torn tissue, grow new tissue, feed critical nerve endings, and nourish any number of other critical bodily processes. In the body of a traditional diabetic, also known as a type I diabetic, this process is derailed because the pancreas is unable to make any insulin. As a result, the bloodstream is flooded with sugar (glucose), which proceeds to wreak havoc on nerve endings while cells are starved for fuel. Only through daily injections of synthetic insulin is the type I diabetic able to survive.

In a type 2 diabetic, the metabolic scenario is somewhat less straightforward. Type 2 diabetics have the same ultimate problem as the type I patient — they are unable to get glucose out of their blood and into their cells — but they arrive at the impasse differently. The pancreas of a type 2 may or may not initially produce enough insulin, but that is almost beside the point. The real culprit in type 2 is a phenomenon called insulin resistance, wherein cells themselves become resistant to insulin's effects. Many believe that such resistance is the result of a defect in the little receptors on the cell surface, those little doorbells. How those receptors get twisted is the matter of much debate. There is evidence, for example, that the trait may be the result of a genetic mutation; "thrifty gene" scholars have even pinpointed a specific allele — or arm — of chromosome 11 as the origin of gene-based insulin resistance. Some populations — African American, Native American, and Mexican American — seem to have this gene in greater percentages than others. Genetics are probably responsible for about 50 percent of the development of insulin resistance.

The other 50 percent likely comes from so-called lifestyle factors, and of all lifestyle factors implicated in insulin resistance, none is more influential than obesity. This is not to say that all obese people are insulin-resistant, or that excess fat alone causes insulin resistance. But obesity certainly makes insulin resistance worse. The mechanism is unclear, but, as the pre-eminent scholar of the phenomenon, Stanford's Gerald Reaven, suggests, it likely relates to the fact that excess visceral fat cells make excess fatty acids, which somehow interfere with the ability of insulin to stimulate the movement of glucose into muscle cells. If you have the least inclination toward insulin resistance, "the more obese you are," Reaven writes, "the more insulin-resistant you will be."

Increasingly, scholars believe that the modern way of eating also causes enhanced insulin resistance. Consider frequent high-energy snacking, which stimulates the pancreas to oversecrete insulin, thereby exposing the liver to longer, uninterrupted bombardment by the hormone. When that happens, according to Victor Zammit, head of cell biology at the Hannah Research Institute in Ayr, Scotland, the liver begins to interpret insulin differently — as a signal to release more fats, in the form of triglycerides, into the bloodstream. Along with the excess insulin (stimulated in the first place by excess snacking) these excess triglycerides tend to make muscle more insulin-resistant. (In the doorbell analogy, it would be as if one constantly rang one's neighbor's doorbell and then ran away; eventually the neighbor would stop coming to the door.) In the final leg of their journey, the triglycerides overload fat cells, where they are supposed to be stored as future energy, and begin to spill over as fatty acids, which in turn strike at the pancreas's insulin-producing beta cells, causing insulin levels to drop and, consequently, blood sugar to spike. That kicks off the dangerous diabetic cycle.

But it is not just how often one eats that can encourage insulin resistance, it's what one eats as well, and in this regard it pays to remember one of the key accomplishments of the Butzian revolution in American food: the commodification of high-fructose corn syrup, the use of which has increased tenfold since Butz's mid-1970s reforms. For years, food technologists and academics alike knew that, in addition to its properties of sweetness and stability (which made it so useful to convenience food makers) there was something else unique about fructose. Unlike its cousin sucrose, fructose is selectively "shunted" toward the liver; it does not go through some of the critical intermediary breakdown steps that sucrose does. This was interesting, but for years no one knew exactly what it meant. Eventually, cell biologists figured out that fructose was being used in the liver as a building block of triglycerides. This it did by mimicking insulin's ability to cause the liver to release fatty acids into the bloodstream (as demonstrated by Zammit in Scotland). Bombarded by fatty acids, muscle tissue develops insulin resistance. Whether humans consume enough high-fructose syrup to activate the effect was something that eluded scientists until the year 2000, when researchers at the University of Toronto in Canada fed a high-fructose diet to Syrian golden hamsters, which have a fat metabolism remarkably similar to that of humans. In weeks, the hamsters developed high triglyceride levels and insulin resistance.

Preliminary human studies also indict concentrated fructose. Two years ago, the clinical nutritionist John Bantle at the University of Minnesota at Minneapolis fed two dozen healthy volunteers a diet that derived 17 percent of total calories from fructose — the percentage that Bantle believes about 27 million Americans eat regularly (particularly all of those fast-food "heavy users" and drinkers of 32-ounce Cokes). Bantle then measured the volunteers' blood fats and sugars, and then switched them to a diet sweetened mainly with sucrose. The results were dramatic. The fructose diet produced significantly higher triglycerides in the blood — in men about 32 percent higher — than the sucrose-sweetened diet. The fructose diets also made triglyceride levels peak faster — just after the meal, when such fats can do the most damage to artery walls. To put a point on such observations, the conservative *American Journal of Clinical Nutrition* published one article that bluntly (and uncharacteristically) concluded that "these deleterious changes [by dietary fructose] occur in the absence of *any* beneficial effect . . . and these abnormalities . . . appear to be greater in those individuals already at an increased risk for coronary artery disease."

The fructose trouble hardly ends there. Fructose consumption — it now constitutes 9 percent of the average individual's daily energy intake (and up to 20 percent of the average child's diet) —

has lately prompted science to look at another, more controversial, theory — that fructose consumption *itself* may have led to increased rates of obesity, not merely through increased calories, but through a variety of complex chemical reactions it stimulates in the human body. The theory has its origins in the 1970s, when European researchers began to chart the exact cellular pathways that determine whether or not a cell burns or stores new fuel. They soon focused on two critical enzymes, acyl-CoA and acyl-carnitine, which act as pathway regulators on the cell surface. Both seem to "tell" the inner cell whether to "store" or "burn" a newly arriving fat particle. Scientists then looked at the effect of different fats and sugars on these enzymes. Two elements, glycerol and fructose, emerged as principal players. When these were present in abundance, acyl-CoA and acyl-carnitine levels were depressed, thus leading the researchers to conclude that fructose and glycerol "lower the rate of fatty acid oxidation." For almost a decade however, such work was virtually ignored by American nutritional scientists, who were much more interested in dietary fats rather than dietary sugars. This was largely because the research agenda had been set by the American Heart Association, which had decided that dietary fat was the principal cause of excess, artery-clogging cholesterol.

Then, in the late 1990s, things began to change. One factor was the sheer magnitude and frequency of fructose consumption, mainly in new convenience foods, pastries, and snacks. The connection with obesity grew when, in 1999, the *American Journal of Clinical Nutrition* published a revealing graph, showing, on one axis, the rate of growth of new food products (principally fructose-laden convenience foods, snacks, and candy), and, on the other axis, the rate of growth of the average national BMI. Both rates increased across the same span of years at almost exactly the same incline. More research followed. Older research was revived and given a second look. A 1993 study from the U.K. showed another pathway and mechanism implicating fructose and obesity. Reviewing studies of animal and human models, the

University of London veterinary scientist P. A. Mayes narrated how fructose consumption led to increased production in the liver of an enzyme called pyruvate dehydrogenase, or PDH. PDH is another chemical gateway that tells a cell whether to burn fatty acids or sugars; the more that is present at the cell surface, the more the cell will tend to burn sugar instead of fat. "Long-term absorption of fructose," Mayes concluded, "causes enzyme adaptations that increase lipogenesis [fat formation] and VLDL [bad cholesterol] formation, leading to triglyceridemia [too many triglycerides in the blood], decreased glucose tolerance, and hyperinsulinemia [too much insulin in the blood]." By 1995 a farsighted team of researchers from the University of California at Berkeley, studying how certain sugars alter how the body selects fuels to burn, concluded basically the same thing: Longterm dietary changes involving simple sugars — as had happened in two decades with fructose — "contribute to [overall] changes in fat oxidation." Overuse of fructose, these and other studies were saying, was skewing the national metabolism toward fat storage.

Still, nutritionists involved in public health pronouncements remained reluctant to single out one specific kind of sugar; most of their careers had been made, after all, in demonizing dietary fat. Nonetheless, in 2001, one high-visibility group from the Department of Medicine at Children's Hospital in Boston took the leap. In a brilliant methodological tactic, researchers under Dr. David Ludwig singled out childhood consumption of soda pop and obesity as their target. Soda is, ninety-nine out of a hundred times, nothing but high-fructose corn syrup and carbonated water, with a few flavoring agents thrown in for brand distinction. The researchers tracked 548 ethnically diverse Massachusetts schoolchildren (average age eleven) for nineteen months, looking at the association between their weight at the beginning of the study, intake of soda, and weight at the end of the study period. The results were revealing. For one thing, 57 percent increased their intake over the nineteen-month period. The calories from just one extra soft drink a day gave a child a 60 percent greater chance of becoming obese. One could even link specific amounts of soda to specific amounts of weight gain. Each daily drink added .18 points to a child's BMI. This, the researchers noted, was *regardless of what else they ate or how much they exercised.* "Consumption of sugar[HFCS]-sweetened drinks," they concluded, "is associated with obesity in children."

The reaction by the food industry was predictable, with many of its underwritten scientific advisory boards issuing proclamations that fructose was a natural product of Mother Nature. It was, they inevitably pointed out, made from good old American corn. But none of those organizations has yet refuted the growing scientific concern that, when all is said and done, fructose — as produced by modern food processors and used by the American consumer — is about the furthest thing from natural that one can imagine, let alone eat.

Although not as intensively studied as fructose, palm oil and palm kernel oil, the other great legacies (along with cheap soybean oil) of the Butz years, have also rendered their share of obesity-related woes. Both are implicated in insulin resistance. As saturated fats — fats rich in fatty acids — both tend to raise total and LDL, or "bad," cholesterol, thereby contributing to atherosclerosis and coronary heart disease. (A highly publicized campaign in the late 1980s by the businessman Ira Sokolow against the use of palm oil for french-frying led to a marked decrease in usage.) Palm oil's impact on insulin effectiveness, on its ability to stimulate glucose use by cells, is less clear. One study by researchers in the Netherlands demonstrated that palm oil was only half as effective as sunflower seed oil in fostering glucose uptake. In another study by the same group, groups of lab rats were fed diets containing different kinds of oils (sunflower seed oil, palm oil, olive oil, linseed oil, cocoa butter, and coconut oil). The researchers then looked at the level of insulin response by fat cells in each group. The result: Compared to the other oils, cocoa butter, coconut oil, and palm oil were negatively correlated to insulin response. No one can yet tell if this effect is due to something particular to all tropical oils, or if the effect is simply a reaction to all saturated fats, but one thing is certain: There are far better fats and oils to use as an industrial oil than palm oil and its relatives. Which is certainly something to keep in mind as palm oil's proponents attempt, as they have recently, to revive its use by promoting its "healthful" amounts of vitamin A.

Regardless of how one arrives at his or her insulin resistance — and there are an estimated 60 million Americans who have it — the path that follows the condition is almost always a painful one, eventually leading to full-blown type 2 diabetes. And because insulin resistance often goes undetected — the pancreas can delay its main effects by pumping out extra insulin before eventually wearing out its capacity to do so — one may be suffering from near–type 2 damage long before the condition is officially diagnosed. Too much sugar in the blood becomes the catalyst for a dirge of woes that can eventually render the sufferer all but helpless.

The obese diabetic may first notice strange things happening to his or her feet; they may tingle, or they may be numb. When they are bruised or scratched, they may take a long time to heal. This is because excess sugar in the blood has damaged vital nerve endings and, in the worst case, caused atherosclerosis, leading to reduced blood flow to the limbs. The consequent numbness can mask a severe injury, which can become infected, eventually leading to gangrene and amputation. This happens more often than one might suspect, particularly as the disease progresses into middle and late middle age.

Now move up the legs. Behind the knees one may develop *Acanthosis nigricans,* the dark, velvety patches that Dr. Kaufman saw on young Jason. Too much insulin in the blood causes that. Muscle tissue on the calves and thighs, starved of fuel because it has become so insulin-resistant, may atrophy. The diabetic may, then, be losing muscle as he or she gains fat, the worst of all possible situations.

It is likely, however, that the obese diabetic will be preoccu-

pied with other, more painful woes. Because the obese tend to ex-
crete excess cholesterol, they are also more likely to form gallstones. In adult women, obesity raises the chances of contracting
such twofold. In children, obesity accounts for somewhere between 8 and 33 percent of gallstones. This may seem like a rather
abstract development — until the body decides to pass the stones,
causing biliary colic. In that case, as the *Merck Manual* puts it,
there is nothing abstract about it at all: "In contrast to other types
of colic, biliary colic is constant, with pain progressively rising to
a plateau and falling gradually, lasting up to several hours. Nausea and vomiting are often associated." Elsewhere in the abdomen, the obese diabetic may contract liver steatosis — fatty liver
disease. Although by itself not life-threatening, fatty livers have
been shown to lead to tissue scarring and eventually to cirrhosis,
particularly if the patient continues to gain weight. Obese children are also at risk for steatohepatitis, with the most severe cases
leading, again, to cirrhosis.

Menstrual and other sex hormone–related conditions increase
in proportion to weight too. Obese girls tend to experience earlier
menarche, often before age ten. As one ages, obesity can incul-
cate patterns of late or absent menstruation. About 40 to 60 percent of adult women who contract polycystic ovary syndrome —
large but benign ovarian cysts — are overweight or obese. The
syndrome often brings with it acne, *Acanthosis nigricans,* and
hirsutism (excess hairiness), the latter in such abundance as to require its own regimen of treatment.

Excess blood sugar and insulin continue to damage other parts
of the body. For the same reasons that high blood sugar causes
foot problems, it causes numbness in hands, arms, and legs. Then
there are the eyes, perhaps the most delicate of diabetes' targets.
With the disease out of control, and with a bad diet repeatedly
jacking up blood sugar and blood fat levels, blood sugar damages
the small blood vessels of the retina, the part of the eye that is
sensitive to light. The broken vessels can leak blood into the eyes,
form deposits, and/or cause the retina to grow new, much more

fragile vessels, which bleed even more easily. When they begin to bleed into the vitreous humor (a clear, jelly-like substance that fills the center of the eye) the obese diabetic will get blurred vision, leading to double vision and, eventually, blindness. About 80 percent of people who have diabetes for fifteen years or more have some damage to blood vessels in the retina.

Numb limbs, darkened skin, painful gallstones, hair sprouting from embarrassing places, fading vision — such is the lot of the obese diabetic. And that is just the beginning, for any biography of an obese body would not be complete without chapters on nondiabetic medical consequences. Even if one does not become a full-blown diabetic, insulin resistance, combined with an ongoing poor diet and too many visceral fat cells, can lead to the triple threat of coronary artery disease (CAD), hypertension, and stroke.

CAD proceeds directly from atherosclerosis, a thickening of the artery walls due to the repeated presence of lipids — blood fats; these come from diet, but are also multiplied via the insulin-resistant patient's propensity to produce too much compensatory insulin, which in turn sparks the liver to spew fatty acids into the bloodstream. (A new study shows that structural changes in the artery walls that lead to hardening begin as early as age twelve.) Hypertension — high blood pressure due to constricted blood vessels — has more complex and still many unknown causes, but two emergent theories, again put forth by Stanford's Gerald Reaven, go something like this: First, hyperinsulinemia causes the kidneys to retain salt and water, thereby boosting total blood volume and its consequent pressure against artery walls. Next come changes in the blood vessels themselves. Here insulin plays the pivotal role again. Because the hormone acts on the central nervous system, it can encourage the arteries to decrease in diameter. Insulin also catalyzes the action of catecholamines, which act, in part, to decrease the diameter of blood vessels, again pushing up blood pressure. (Hypertension is nine times more frequent in obese children; 20 percent of obese children between five and eleven already have it.) With clotted, constricted, and overloaded arteries, the stage is set for all kinds of vascular mischief, one of the most deadly of which is stroke. Stroke happens when all of these conditions cause the vessels of the human brain to become blocked, depriving the organ of much needed oxygen and nutrients and causing it, eventually, to cease functioning.

The brain suffers from obesity in other ways too, responding with a condition known as *Pseudotumor cerebri*. As the name suggests, this is a brain tumor–like condition caused when excess abdominal weight presses down upon the lungs and the heart, causing increased pressure on the vein returning blood from the brain. The most common symptoms are headaches, vomiting, blurred vision, and double vision. Obesity occurs in 30 to 80 percent of children with pseudotumor. The chances of a child getting the condition increase by twenty times when body weight exceeds 20 percent above the ideal.

Then there are the orthopedic problems. First comes the obvious: arthritic joints caused by simply carrying too much weight. Next is a condition known as slipped capital femoral epiphysis — a slipped hip. Obese children succumb to it much more often, and at substantially younger ages, than the nonobese. Its consequences can be painful and chronic and eventually require surgical insertion of a screw in the hip. The same can be said of Blount's disease, also known as *Tibia vara*. In Blount's, the legs respond to early weight excess by becoming bowed, and contrary to popular conceptions about bowed legs, this is not merely a cosmetic inconvenience. Consider a recent case report, detailed by J. Richard Bower, the chief of orthopedic surgery at the Alfred I. Du Pont Institute: "The patient is a 14 and one half year old black male with a one year history of worsening left knee pain. He states that the pain began in both knees and was intermittent. . . . Over the past six months the pain is more isolated to the left knee and has become constant in nature. Within the past two weeks the constant pain has become bad enough to limit his activities. He is unable to attend school or walk more than several hundred feet because of the pain. The pain is now affecting his sleep. . . . The adolescent is morbidly obese." As are 80 percent of children with Blount's.

Now drones the true dirge of the obese child — respiratory diseases. These come in three forms. The first, Pickwickian syndrome, is named after the ever somnolent Joe the Fat Boy in Dickens's *Pickwick Papers.* The syndrome starts when large amounts of abdominal fat cause the child to breathe in a rapid, shallow fashion, with increasing intervals of breathlessness. This leads to oxygen deprivation, chronic sleepiness, and, if untreated, heart failure. Excess fat tissue in the throat and uvula is also the direct cause of obstructive sleep apnea in obese children, a third of whom display the main symptoms of apathy, listlessness, nighttime sleeplessness, and daytime somnolence. More troubling are the condition's effects on learning. According to a report in the *International Journal of Obesity,* "Obese children with obstructive sleep apnea demonstrate clinically significant decrements in learning and memory function."

Lastly there is the condition known as allergic asthma. For the past three decades, epidemiologists have watched a progressive rise in this wheezing condition, particularly among children between five and eighteen. The two principal theories about its origin — increased time spent around or near indoor allergens and the rise in childhood antibiotic use — have recently been joined by a new theory of causation: the general decline in childhood physical activity. In this scenario, lack of the strengthening effects of exercise leads to weakened lungs, making it easier for wheezing reactions to set in. A study by the Respiratory Sciences Center at the University of Arizona showed that females who became overweight or obese between six and eleven years of age were seven times more likely to develop new asthma symptoms than those who were normal weight.

Obesity makes for special problems when fat girls grow up to become fat mothers. Women who are overweight or obese before becoming pregnant are much more likely to develop gestational diabetes and hypertension of pregnancy, also known as pre-eclampsia; they will inevitably need longer and more intensive hospitalization. A mother's excessive pre-pregnancy weight also greatly increases her chances of having a baby that is stillborn or that will die shortly after birth. If the child survives, he or she is 30 to 40 percent more likely to present with a variety of birth defects, ranging from spina bifida to heart malformations to defects in the abdominal wall. Folic acid supplements are less likely to prevent such defects in the offspring of the obese, who are at increased risk of becoming obese themselves, thereby setting in motion the vicious cycle once more.

As if all of this were not enough, the obese child who becomes an obese adult will also have an increased risk of cancer. In early 2001 the American Cancer Society, after years of deliberation, issued a special statement on the connection in its annual *Cancer Facts and Figures*. Obesity, the society declared, was "linked to an increased risk of breast cancer after menopause and to cancer of the endometrium, ovaries, colon, prostate and gall bladder." Again, much of the problem derives from excess visceral fat cells, which, among other things, play a key role in converting estrogen to estradiol, a more active form of the hormone that can promote tumor growth. If the obese individual is insulin-resistant, compensatory oversecretion of insulin will cause overproduction of insulin-like growth factor, related, in turn, to growth factors that bring about colon, breast, and prostate cancer. Cancer, the obsession of twentieth-century medicine, has entered the new millennium as the special burden of the obese.

As Fran Kaufman had observed, something had indeed changed.

Outside of the medical consequences to the individual, what are the economic consequences to the nation if obesity is merely incorporated into the American way of life rather than resisted?

There are, first and foremost, the premature deaths of more than 280,000 Americans every year, the figure the American

Medical Association now believes reflects the number of obesity-related mortalities. There is the $100 billion annual price tag for the care and treatment of diabetics, the majority of new cases being a direct result of excess weight. That boils down to one in every ten dollars dedicated to health care. In terms of federal resources, diabetes alone commands one in every four Medicare dollars. These are considered to be conservative estimates. Most policy experts on the subject believe that diabetes is subject to the classic epidemiological "rule of halves"; because of its overwhelming residence at lower social addresses, and because one can have the disease for long periods of time without feeling sick, only half of all diabetics are ever diagnosed. Of those, only half are ever treated. And of those only half ever have their disease managed effectively.

Obesity takes its toll on our daily quality of life too. Between 1988 and 1994 the number of days of lost work due to obesity increased by 50 percent — to 39 million days, worth $3.9 billion. There were also 239 million restricted activity days due to obesity, 89.5 million bed rest days, and 62.6 million physician visits, the last equivalent to an 88 percent rise over 1988. As A. M. Wolfe and G. A. Colditz of the University of Virginia concluded in a study of such costs among a population of 88,000 U.S. residents, "The economic and personal health costs of overweight and obesity are enormous and *compromise the health of the United States*" (emphasis added). As a recent RAND/University of Chicago report noted, "More Americans are obese than smoke, use illegal drugs, or suffer from ailments unrelated to obesity."

How will the average person feel obesity's economic pinch? To figure that out, four researchers from the independent Policy Analysis Inc. (PAI) set up a sophisticated model of a hypothetical HMO with 1 million members. Using reference data from a large managed health care plan in the Pacific Northwest, the researchers then projected the number of cases of eight diseases for which obesity is an established risk factor (coronary heart disease, hypertension, hypercholesterolemia, gall bladder disease, stroke, type 2 diabetes, osteoarthritis of the knee, and endometrial cancer). The results were mind-boggling, even to jaded public health types. In a population of 1 million, the PAI researchers found, "obesity would account for 132,900 cases of hypertension (45 percent of all cases), 58,500 cases of type 2 diabetes (85 percent), 51,000 cases of hypercholesterolemia (18 percent), and 16,500 cases of coronary heart disease (35 percent)." The total costs of obesity to the HMO? $345.9 million annually, or 41 percent of the total for the eight diseases studied — "substantial," as the researchers put it.

And what will happen when people who take care of themselves start to understand why their own health care bill keeps skyrocketing? "We believe the effect will be like that of second-hand smoke," says James O. Hill, of the University of Colorado and the dean of American obesity studies. "When people who are fit really begin to understand this, it will be a catalyst for one of two things, though likely both: anger, and then a demand for change." Hill has been studying the phenomenon in Pueblo, Colorado, where groups of patients, health providers, academics, physicians, and policy makers are trying to come up with a way to involve HMOs more directly in treating and preventing obesity. "The main thing we see is real shock when people digest this. They get very worked up — and why not? They are taking care of themselves. But they also want to know: What can we do besides just throw more money at this?"

One approach would be for HMOs to get more proactively involved in identifying obesity-related problems within their contracted populations. An enlightened HMO might sponsor a free blood sugar testing clinic, with employees who test high being counseled to schedule more complete workups in the future. But what then? Not a few fat people's rights organizations would argue that such an approach would merely legitimize discrimination against the obese, giving them a medical stigma to go with their aesthetic stigma. (Yes, this may sound crazy, but such concerns are a fact of life in large organizations, particularly large governmental organizations, where obesity rates run particularly high.) Moreover, mainstream (read: middle) America remains in deep denial about obesity; it will likely be some time until the culture connects the proverbial dots and demands such testing. As Gerry Oster, one of the authors of the PAI study, says, "We have a long long way to go until the average person gets a clue about the connection. I am not representative at all of the typical attitude toward obesity. None of my friends are obese; we are coastal professionals involved in health care research. But go to the Mall of America in Minneapolis — I'd bet the obesity rate you see there is 75 percent or more." A culture that condones obesity, whether consciously or unconsciously, undermines any attempts to convince people to pare down.

Yet not taking such basic preventive measures merely encourages more rampant obesity, which, in turn, fuels its own kind of social sorting, one based on both aesthetics and social class. The aspiring classes of the country tilt toward thinness as a social goal. Perusing the pages of any "New Economy" magazine of the 1990s, one was pressed to find a single example of an obese CEO, let alone an obese venture capitalist. Ditto today's heroes in *Fortune* or *Forbes*. The operative notion is simple: If one can't control one's own contours, how can one be trusted to control someone else's money?

Even the Clinton-Lewinsky scandal had a strong taint of upper-class anti-fatism to it. As Jane Gallop, a distinguished professor of English at the University of Wisconsin at Milwaukee, commented in the *New York Times,* "There's a moment in the Barbara Walters interview where Monica relates that he [Clinton] would always leave his shirt untucked because of his belly, and you just feel that was one of the ways where Monica and Bill get connected. If the right wing in this country is still really moralistic about sex, the left is moralistic about food — that's where the new style of moralism about control is. Well-educated people are supposed to be in control of the amount of body fat they have.

The people who are disgusted by Clinton's fat and by Monica's aren't the right wing, they're the ones who wanted a yuppie president with the right amount of body fat at the helm."

Although one might quibble with her left-right dialectics (after all, it is George W. Bush who has the right body fat, not to mention a pulse lower than that of Seabiscuit), Gallop clearly is on to one thing: When it comes to fat, the affluent are afraid. Very afraid. They will do anything not to be affiliated with it. In the upper classes, fat is seen as the great cheat — a barrier to performance, a denier of rewards delayed, a mark of the uncontrolled, primal fellow supposedly left behind in the individual's arduous upward economic march. To be affiliated with being fat would put the affluent person on the wrong side of the stigma, where the dynamic would seem to cut the other way — fat attracting fat.

Fat attracting fat! Johannes Hebebrand, the German psychiatrist who was so taken aback by how unashamed obese Americans seem to be, has been studying that side of the stigma for more than a decade. "We got very interested in this area some time ago, when we saw that negative impressions about fat people — as indicated in various surveys and attitude tests — showed a huge jump in just ten years. It led us to ask: If people feel stigmatized, will they be more likely to mate with other stigmatized people, in this case other fat people?" he says. "The other factor was the huge jump in the obesity rate itself, and the fact that everyone was saying it had to be entirely an environmental issue, because twenty years was too short of a time for genetic mutations to appear. We started to think that maybe that was not entirely true. Maybe environment — via assortative mating — was accelerating genetic expression of obesity."

To find out if that were the case, Hebebrand and his fellows at the University of Marburg, Germany, examined the parents of 471 extremely obese children and adolescents. The researchers took down three key pieces of data: the parents' current measured height, the parents' current self-measured height, *and the parents' recalled weights and heights at ages twenty and thirty, the period when most couples meet and marry.* They then referenced these measures against BMI averages for the general population. When they charted the cross-references, they found a high degree of assortative mating; obese children tended to have parents who mated when they themselves were obese. Although the results are only suggestive — Hebebrand was unable to show that the rate of assortative mating itself has increased over time — his finding falls in line with what is already known about obese children and obese parents. It is this: Obese parents influence their children's fatness both through genetics and through environment. "It is not exactly a straight line," Hebebrand says. "There are all kinds of other factors going on here. Take the case of the thinner person marrying the fatter person, who soon drags the thinner person down into his or her habits. He watches ten hours of TV and she begins to do the same, and over time she becomes obese too. In this case it was not the genetic expression of obesity from assortative mating that makes for fat kids. It's the environment that *both* the parents produce."

In all of this — fat attracting fat, stigma causing assortative mating, fat producing fat — there glimmers just a touch of the old eugenicist impulse. Yet in this case, recognizing such a dynamic might help prevent a eugenic reality, for however parents become obese, one thing is indisputable: Fat parents are more likely — much more likely — to raise fat children, who are in turn more likely to be fat adults, who are then more likely to continue the daisy chain until, as James Hill fears, all Americans are overweight or obese. And that day is not far away . . .

Let us now spend an imaginary day with a typical American, circa 2050, when overweight and obesity are the norm, and when the social divisions are not between the slim and the fat but between the obese and the not so obese. In other words, a lot like today, only intensified by a factor of one hundred.

Our average guy arises late in the morning, later than he had planned. He has slept poorly. The night before, the CPAP (for continuously pressurized air pathway) machine that provides an extra forceful flow of air to aid with his sleep apnea had been louder than usual. Looking in the mirror, he takes in his visage: Across the bridge of his nose and under his eyes rises a freshet of new acne, the nightly legacy of the sticky plastic face mask he must wear in order to remain hooked up to the CPAP machine. "Shit," he mutters.

He takes a shower, shaves, dresses. He curses at his ever too small pants and shirt — hadn't he just purchased a larger size a few months ago? — and then turns to the mirror again. He examines the dark circles under his eyes and the *Acanthosis nigricans* on his neck, then decides to cover up the latter with his wife's face powder. From his desk he picks up his blood sugar meter and, in the first of a half-dozen tests he will administer throughout the day, pricks his finger, draws blood, and measures his glucose level. He then injects his thigh with the first of several doses of insulin. Running late, he decides that, despite the worsening pain in his arthritic knee, he will forgo his pain medication, and walks out to the kitchen.

He cannot have his favorite breakfast, pancakes, because his blood sugar will soar if he eats more than one. (And what is the use of that? he reasons.) He drinks a cup of black coffee, has some oatmeal with nonfat milk and artificial sweetener, kisses his wife, and leaves for work.

In traffic, his blood pressure soars. Did he take the medication for that today? He cannot remember. The cell phone beeps; it is his wife reminding him that he has to take his son Jonny to the endocrinologist today. Only nine, the boy is already forty pounds overweight, and just last week he had another fainting spell at recess. It may have been from hypoglycemia. Whatever the cause, the school nurse sent home an embarrassing ultimatum: Get Jonny checked or she would have to notify social services.

Finally our average guy arrives at work. The office is humming; business is good. But, again, the new sales charts underscore that, as a salesman, our man is not what he used to be. Getting in and out of the car to make sales calls, always arduous even when he was not obese, is now something to be avoided altogether. The two-hour drop in his afternoon energy level doesn't exactly help either. Nor does his aching knee. He checks his blood sugar and begins the afternoon round of phone calls. He is glad that he ordered the large-type phone pad, since his eyesight too is not what it once was.

At around four, a marked silence falls outside his office door. His officemates burst in with a birthday cake and a song. His assistant gets out a knife and begins serving slices of the cake with ice cream. She offers him a plate, and he demurs. She insists. He refuses again, but feels ashamed to reveal why he cannot eat such a sugary treat, and so eventually relents. An hour later he is flushed, sweaty, and dizzy. He vows never to do such a stupid thing again.

Outside, the cool air dries his sweat-beaded brow. He gets in his car and drives over to day care to pick up Jonny. When he gets there his son is crying. "They . . . they used me as a dodgeball target again!" he explains. "They . . . they call me earthquake boy because I'm so . . ." Jonny doesn't need to finish the sentence.

"Aren't there other . . . *heavy* kids in your class? What do they do when . . ."

His son cuts him off. "It's just that I'm the biggest," he blurts out.

It is a long, uncomfortable drive.

At the doctor's, the boy fares better than he thought he would. "I'm thinking that the fainting may be more from stress — from all the teasing and harassment — than from his blood sugar," the doctor says. "But you better get that hip checked out . . . When did he start walking like that?" He writes out a referral to a specialist in pediatric bone disease. "Just in case," he says, not very convincingly.

At home, waiting for dinner, he opens the mail. There is a notice from his HMO — again — telling him that his rates have gone up. Again. Also, the co-pay for medications has jumped; given the fact that he pays upward of $200 in co-payments a month already, it makes him worry: What would he do if he ever lost his job, or even if the company scaled back its health coverage? He shudders to recall a nightmare he had earlier in the week, one in which he was being told by his physician that "amputating today is not what it used to be — amputees can live full, long lives . . ." He decides to pay more attention to the chronic numbness in his left foot.

Dinner, since it is diabetically correct, is not worth eating, but he does so anyway, if just to spend some time with his wife. She, too, has weight-related woes; though not yet a full-blown diabetic, she nonetheless feels the limitations of being obese. Her energy level is low. She seems to sweat endlessly. Her gynecologist has called her back for more x-rays and a discussion of whether she should have surgery to remove the large but (so far) benign ovarian cyst she has had for the past two years.

Later, while the family is watching TV, he sneaks into the kitchen and eats handful after handful of the cookies he stashed behind the coffee tin the evening before. The momentary pleasure is followed by a rush of guilt, then nausea, then clammy sweating. He relaxes for a while longer, resolves never to do *that* again, and decides to turn in early.

In bed, he sets the CPAP machine on low, puts in his earplugs so he doesn't have to listen to the thing chug and puff all night, and gets ready to put on the mask. Shit, he thinks. Perhaps if he swabs it with alcohol first he will not wake up with another crop of unsightly red zits.

They are, after all, more than a little embarrassing, particularly at age thirty-five.

7

·····················

WHAT CAN BE DONE

BOUT FIVE YEARS AGO, the schools of San Antonio, Texas, some of the most rapidly growing in the nation, confronted a troubling revelation: A new study by a local nonprofit health agency showed that, unless administrators acted to make substantial changes, there would soon be as many as 3000 type 2 diabetic children in the district's fifty elementary schools. The principal cause, the study had concluded, was excess body weight. Almost all of the children at risk had BMIs of greater than 27 — they were already substantially overweight — and many had BMIs far in excess of 30, the cutoff for clinical obesity. Nearly as awful — at least to the men and women who ran the schools — was the implication that the San Antonio schools were themselves at least partly to blame for the trend. The study authors — all from the local Social and Health Research Center, headed by Dr. Robert Trevino — had found, among other things, that the school cafeterias were serving a menu laced with excess fats and sugars, that the food service staff had no idea about how to make fresh fruits and produce palatable to kids, that after-school care was bereft of any meaningful physical activity, and that teachers in the districts had few if any classroom materials for teaching sound nutrition and exercise practices. "We scared the hell out of them," says Trevino of the school

155

district's reaction to his study. "They realized it was both the right thing to do *and* that it was in their self-interest to deal with it."

The annals of public health are chock-full of such momentary bureaucratic realizations — realizations that soon dim and fade as new and seemingly more urgent concerns wrinkle the public brow. The course that usually follows is as predictable as a Hollywood B movie: Posters inveighing against the evil get tacked up around the school. Memos go out to teachers, principals, and sometimes even parents. There follows a special "awareness" program, designed to change attitudes toward the problem and invite candid discussion. More pamphlets will be passed out. The PTA might receive a special report on the subject. An already overburdened principal will be assigned to head a committee to look into possible solutions. The issue will take its place alongside the others waiting in line, collecting administrative dust.

History, however, will in this case take due note: This is exactly what San Antonio did not do. Instead, the school district tried an aggressive and unconventional strategy that broke the mold of the traditional public health response to chronic disease. The first part of the strategy was to recognize that obesity and type 2 diabetes among its students was, first and foremost, a class issue. It wasn't something that, as most public health campaigns (often artificially) insist, affects everybody. "It's not a gene thing, it's a poverty thing," as Trevino says. That observation guided the district's allocation of resources — time, money, and expertise — and, as a result, made for a more targeted, efficient solution.

The second part of San Antonio's approach was even more controversial. Instead of focusing the main part of its efforts on the children themselves, the administration turned its attention to changing itself. "We didn't believe it was enough to put a few more dollars into a nutrition class and so to change some kids' attitudes and beliefs about food and health," says Trevino, who was put in charge of the effort. "We believed that you had to change their environment — their total school environment."

This Trevino and his staff did by devising an extensive series of lesson plans designed to change the health environments of targeted elementary schools. In the cafeteria, food service workers were tutored in state-of-the-art food preparation and food presentation schemes — all designed to increase the amounts of fruits and vegetables consumed and to lessen the amounts of added fats and sugars. Older students were drafted to monitor the eating habits of their younger schoolmates at lunchtime. In classrooms, students had new lesson plans designed to educate them about what choices they should make in the cafeteria setting — in essence, creating demand for the new cafeteria fare. Trevino also dedicated thirty-two new lesson plans to after-school care, where TV and video games had come to supplant physical activity as the recreational mainstay. The result was to transform the traditional after-school program into a highly popular "health club" — a place where child care met both traditional and nontraditional exercise and sports programs. There were even lesson plans for parents, principals, and school medical personnel.

A year later, the district assessed Trevino's intervention. In the cafeteria, there had been two dramatic improvements. Compared with a control group of schools that had not adopted the changes, the percentage of calories from fat dropped from an average of 34 percent to 30 percent — well in line with USDA guidelines — and the number of fruits and vegetables consumed per meal had more than doubled, from 1.2 to 2.5. The control group's fat content and fruit and vegetable consumption remained the same. Fitness scores, mainly aerobic capacity, also improved dramatically in the experimental schools, rising by 4.6 percent against the control group's rise of .8 percent. Most important, the average blood sugar measurement among the schools' type 2 diabetics had registered remarkable decreases — from 123 to 99; the kids in the experimental schools now had near-normal blood glucose counts.

San Antonio's success points up one of the few bright patches in Fatland America: By and large, we already know what kind of basic health strategies work, at least when it comes to children, and, in many cases, what works for adults, when it comes to reducing both the incidence of obesity and its consequences. It was not always so. In a review published in 1978, researchers gloomily concluded that "clinically significant changes for obese children are rare. Follow-up data . . . show consistently that subjects fail to continue losing weight or even maintain weight losses experienced during treatment." By 1994 the general wisdom on the subject had completely reversed itself, with one reviewer noting that "overall, treatments for childhood and adolescent obesity were found to produce medium sized treatment effects at posttest" with follow-ups showing that they "continue to maintain moderate results." Basic behavioral modification was the treatment of choice.

It is hardly surprising that the two most important behavioral changes involve food and exercise — less of one and more of the other. It is surprising, however, just how much of a difference such changes can make. Numerous recent studies — across large numbers of diverse Americans, as well as studies from other countries — show not only that the effects of type 2 diabetes can be substantially reduced through better eating and vigorous exercise, but that diseases like type 2 can actually be prevented by adopting such behaviors. In one study sponsored by the National Institute of Diabetes and Digestive and Kidney Diseases released in 2001, researchers from Massachusetts General Hospital recruited 3300 people with a condition known as impaired glucose tolerance — a kind of precursor to type 2 in which the body's ability to process sugar is slowed, but without any outward symptoms of disease. The subjects were then split up into three groups. One received a daily dose of metformin, a common pharmaceutical treatment for diabetes, along with basic dietary and exercise advice. A second group received a placebo along with the same advice. The third group got no drug, but instead received regular coaching on how to incorporate exercise into their daily schedules and how to best modify their diets. Three years later, the results were published. Among participants receiving the placebo, 11 percent developed diabetes. Among those receiving metformin, 7.8 percent developed the disease — a reduction of about one third. The big surprise was what happened among those who got no drug but who received in-depth coaching on diet and exercise. Among that group, only 4.8 percent developed diabetes — about half the rate of the control group. Among those in the coached group who were aged sixty or older, the drop in the disease rate was even more precipitous — nearly three quarters. In fact, in one third of the group, blood glucose levels returned to normal. The message was clear: Simple, consistent changes in diet and activity levels can dramatically alter an individual's metabolic destiny.

The key qualifier is the term "consistent." Getting that consistency comes with a price. In the case of the study that price was an investment in time and resources — weekly classes, coaches who followed a participant's progress, continuing medical and dietary monitoring by committed professionals. The question from a broader, policy-oriented point of view seems clear: How can we encourage such investments by large numbers of individuals, so that they become habit? The answer can be found in a number of programs that are dealing successfully with children who are either obese or at risk of becoming so. In other words, with the potentially obese adults of the future.

For twenty years, the trailblazer in the arena of childhood obesity treatment has been Stanford University's Leonard Epstein. A pediatrician and the head of the Stanford Pediatric Weight Control Program, Epstein pioneered the use of basic behavioral modification techniques, combined with a special diet and exercise program, to treat obesity in young children. The cornerstone of his approach is what he has dubbed the Stoplight Diet, which defines all foods by their calorie content and then divides them up into the three colors of the traffic light: red (for stop), yellow (for proceed with caution), and green (eat as one pleases). Children then count up the number of servings of each "color" so as to monitor their daily calorie count. This kind of clear, unambiguous division has been crucial, says Epstein. "It is our experience that some patients find looking for loopholes to be challenging and rewarding. As a result, it is better to leave little room for interpretation in defining dietary changes." He also notes that low-fat or diet versions of a normally high-calorie food should be avoided, so as to prevent continued exposure to such tastes.

As one might expect, Epstein is also concerned with increasing a child's physical activity, but his approach swerves from the predictable paths in two important ways. First, though Epstein believes that both structured exercise — sports and fitness programs — and lifestyle exercise — the "building in of a daily activity like walking to increase one's total expenditure" — can be critical to a child's success in maintaining a healthy weight, he also stresses the importance of activity choice. Children who are allowed to choose their own form of activity seem more likely to meet their daily calorie expenditure goals. Second, Epstein believes that reducing *sedentary* behavior may be more important than promoting physical activity itself. In a series of studies, Epstein and his colleagues at Stanford found that fat children who were either punished for sedentary activities or positively reinforced for decreasing TV viewing, playing computer and board games, or talking on the phone lost significantly more weight than peers who were simply reinforced for increasing physical activity. Epstein speculates about the reason, noting that the children in the decreased sedentary behavior group may have felt more personal control over being more active than those in the other group, who may have felt resentful toward parents who were pushing them into activity.

Epstein has since delineated a number of other elements critical to childhood weight loss programs. They are, in toto, clear, concise, and demanding. Parents must play an active role in treatment, but not necessarily as "co-patients." Rather, they are best used as monitors and enlightened authority figures. They are best left out of specific counseling and exercise sessions, leaving children in a less inhibited arena in which to learn and play. For the first eight to twelve weeks of the program, children should receive weekly follow-up sessions with a counselor; monthly follow-up sessions should continue for the next six to twelve months. In essence, parents are charged with changing the environment that encourages obesity. High-calorie foods should be removed from the home. The number of meals eaten outside the home should be drastically reduced. The soup pot or the casserole dish should be left in the kitchen, not set on the table family style, so as to increase the effort required for additional portions. TVs should be removed from bedrooms. Children should be taught to monitor their body weight, to set reasonable weight loss goals not to exceed one pound a week, and, when required, to enter into a written contract with their parents, with each side carefully delineating their responsibilities in the weight loss effort.

All of which may sound somewhat draconian to the ears of a generation raised to believe that, when it comes to food, personal choice and individual autonomy should trump traditional parental authority. Yet Epstein, unlike a generation of diet gurus who tried to separate control and children's eating habits, can show consistent and healthy results from his approach. Ten years after onset of treatment, some 30 percent of his patients were no longer obese, with 33.5 percent maintaining at least a 20 percent weight loss. His message is unequivocal: Parents must take back control of the table.

Dr. Francine Kaufman, head of the pediatric endocrinology department at Los Angeles's bustling Children's Hospital, has for the last few years successfully woven together some of Epstein's concepts with some of her own to deal with the city's growing problem of childhood type 2 diabetes. Once a week for eight weeks, a group of fifteen or so children, usually accompanied by one parent, file into her department for a two-hour "Kids and Fitness" program. Many come referred by pediatricians, others by school nurses and social services. After a weekly weigh-in, the children and their parents part, the latter to a waiting room, the former to a large conference room. For the next hour, the children are led through a variety of physical activities, ranging from calisthenics to running games to a smaller version of volleyball. "What's amazing is how uninhibited the kids are when the adults are gone and they are just around a bunch of other overweight kids," says Marsha MacKenzie, who runs the program for Kaufman. "The other day we had to laugh, because we asked them what game they would like to play, and a group of them yelled out 'Dodgeball!' Which, of course, they would never do at school, because they are the ones who usually get singled out to be bashed by the ball because they are a natural target for bullies."

For the second hour of Kaufman's program, parents are reunited with their child for a session of nutrition education. It is, to be frank, a troublesome undertaking. During the three sessions I attended, it was not unusual to witness a parent walk into the class eating french fries from McDonald's or sipping a thirty-two-ounce Big Gulp Coke from the local convenience mart. "We have to start from ground zero," says MacKenzie. "It's easy to pass judgment and say, people should know this and people should act this way, but the fact of the matter is that few doctors — let alone parents — know the basics of good nutrition."

MacKenzie and her staff focus each week's discussion on one element of a typical food label — on its fat content, added sugars, calories, portion sizes. Children must then choose from a lineup of typical popular foods, from Cheetos to Cap'n Crunch, and calculate out loud whether it is a good food or a bad food, based on the nutrition information they are studying that week. In a lesson about portions, for example, children were asked first to pour out what they considered one portion. They were then asked to read out loud what the label indicated was one portion, and then to pour out that amount on a small weighing scale. In most cases, the estimated serving size was at least three times the label serving size. "That drives the point home, both for the kids and the parents," says MacKenzie. But it also drives home how much educating needs to be done all over the city.

Schools have long offered tremendous promise as possible battlegrounds against childhood obesity. After all, more than 95 percent of American youth between the ages of five and eighteen are enrolled in school. Though school authority has been whittled down substantially over the years, the institution, by sheer dint of its daily presence, still exerts enormous influence on the lives of its subjects. In the early 1980s the Yale obesity expert Kelly Brownell undertook a small-scale intervention at public schools in Fort Myers, Florida, using nutrition education, physical activity training, changes in food service, and behavior modification techniques with a group of overweight children. The students were able to achieve and sustain a notable weight loss of 15 percent. At the time, many hailed the Brownell approach as a possible new standard in the treatment of childhood obesity.

But the Brownell approach fell victim to the cultural politics of the 1980s, namely, the fear that fat children undergoing such treatment would be stigmatized by their peers. Although it is true that some stigmatizing occurs when any group is singled out for special treatment, this objection — and it was voiced widely and vehemently throughout the decade — ignored the most basic truism about fat and stigmatization: The best way to prevent it is to avoid becoming obese in the first place. As the influential — and, it should be noted, very politically sensitive — *International Journal of Obesity* worried in a review of school programs in 1999, "It is interesting that few studies on school-based treatment of obesity were identified after 1985 . . . Greater awareness of the stigma attached to participating in school-based treatments may have decreased enthusiasm for the programs, *even though they appear to be effective* [emphasis mine]."

Yet the "decreased enthusiasm" seems to be limited to the adults. A more recent survey, based on in-depth interviews with sixty-one overweight adolescents from large inner-city schools, indicated not only that children want such programs, but that they are willing to put up with their possible social ramifications if such a program "was undertaken in a supportive and respectful manner, offered fun activities, was informative, was sensitive to the needs of overweight youth and did not conflict with other activities."

Such interest *by children* has helped launch a new generation of school-based interventions. One of the most promising involves preventive screening. In a study by the University of Houston and Baylor College, scholars looked at how a child's weight in, say, kindergarten would predict that child's chances of becoming obese at a later age. Researchers collated the weights and BMIs of 1013 Mexican American children in a Texas school district. They then tracked the children as they progressed through the system. They found that a kindergarten BMI was highly predictive of obesity at later dates. A child with a low kindergarten BMI of 16.5, for example, would have only a 21 percent chance of becoming obese by fifth grade. A kindergartner with a BMI of 20.9, however, would have a 70 percent chance of becoming an obese fifth grader, while a kindergartner with a BMI of 23.7 would have a 91 percent probability of becoming obese.

While the Houston-Baylor study provides schools with one way to assess a child's relative risks, a program in San Jose, California, has carved a potential path toward reducing both current and future obesity rates. The impetus for it flowed from both theoretical and practical concerns. Researchers from Stanford's Departments of Pediatrics and Medicine had long theorized that if sedentary behaviors like TV-viewing and video game–playing were linked to increased obesity, then programs that taught children to reduce such activities might lead to reductions in adiposity. Meanwhile, teachers and parents in the San Jose School District, aware of increasing obesity rates, were looking for ways to deal with the issue. They decided to give the Stanford researchers access.

To find out if their hypothesis held, the researchers recruited 192 third- and fourth-grade students from two socioeconomically matched schools. One school was assigned to implement a program to reduce TV and video game use, the other was not. The means of the intervention was simple: Limit access to TV sets and game machines, teach children to budget their use, then teach them how to become more selective viewers and players. This the researchers sought to inaugurate and support through traditional classroom instruction. Teachers in the intervention school were trained to administer eighteen specialized lessons, each thirty to fifty minutes in length, taught during regular school hours during the first two months of the school year. The first few lessons taught the students how to monitor and report their own TV and game use, followed by a "TV Turnoff." The TV Turnoff challenged children to watch no TV and play no video games for ten days. After the turnoff, students were told to budget their viewing to seven hours per week. The last lessons sought to increase students' ability to be selective, "intelligent viewers," and to become advocates for reducing the use of such media among their peers. At home, each student TV was equipped with an electronic TV time manager, which logged and measured TV time through the use of a personal code, without which the set would not operate.

The results of the intervention surprised even its most enthusiastic and optimistic supporters. After seven months, TV use in the intervention group was down by one third, compared to the control group. Video game use and viewing of videocassettes were down as well. While not an anticipated outcome, the intervention group also "significantly reduced the frequency of children eating meals in a room with a television turned on." And, most important, children in the intervention group, in the words of the researchers, "had statistically significant relative decreases in BMI, triceps skinfold thickness, waist circumference, and waist to hip ratio." The results did not change with ethnicity or level of parental education.

The success of the San Jose experiment posed an intriguing

question for its authors. Why did the children lose weight? After all, there were no reports that children had dramatically *increased* high-level activity when not watching TV, and when they *were* watching TV their level of snacking matched that of their more sedentary control group. Three answers emerged. One, children in the intervention group snacked less in toto. Two, they had been exposed to dramatically fewer advertisements for high-calorie foods. And three, they likely sought out and engaged in more low-intensity activity. Whatever the cause, the Stanford researchers concluded, reducing TV, video game, and video use "may be a promising, population-based approach to help prevent childhood obesity."

Jim Hill, at the University of Colorado Health Sciences Center, has come to a similar conclusion about larger interventions. As he and John Peters note in a recent issue of *Obesity Reviews,* "The challenge in changing the environment is not to 'go back in time,' but to engineer physical activity and healthy eating back into our lives in a way that is compatible with our socio-cultural value." As Peters and Hill see it, the challenge is to give everyday people the same cognitive tools — essentially a series of goads and rewards — that the more affluent always have had when it comes to managing weight. Hill and his colleagues have launched a program called "Colorado on the Move," a consortium of government agencies, private foundations, educational institutions, and business with one specific, measurable goal: to increase by 2000 steps a day the average number of steps the average Coloradan takes. To do so, they are underwriting the distribution of low-tech step counters around the state. Hill and his colleagues got the idea after comparing the average number of steps daily by an office worker (3000 to 5000) with the average number of steps by people in the National Weight Control Registry (11,000), the most successful single group to maintain weight loss after several years. Beginning with a modest 2000, Colorado on the Move could eventually encourage large numbers of citizens to take increasingly more steps per day. Already some six thousand people are enrolled in pilot programs.

One of the best ways to combat obesity would be to reinvest in traditional public school physical education. Unfortunately, tax-payers have not yet seen fit to do so. (In California in 2001, the legislature was unable to pass even modest legislation that would have funded the creation of written standards for all PE courses in the state.) There is the occasional nod and bow toward the need to "do something" — usually when the ever dismal state fitness test results are published every two years — but there is usually little if any follow-up. Many policy makers believe that today's parents have forever separated school and fitness, preferring either to ignore the subject altogether or to fill their kids' sports cravings through private programs. Unfortunately, that means permanent underfunding of public school PE — the only alternative for the less economically advantaged.

Still, a small core of educators, many of them young PE teachers in some of the nation's most underfunded school districts, have plunged ahead, crafting unique programs specifically targeted at reducing obesity and increasing overall fitness. One of them is Dan Latham, a PE instructor at West Middle School in blue-collar Downey, California. Latham is, in many ways, the kind of fellow that many principals dream about; he is engaging, well-spoken, energetic, and full of ideas — all of which he is convinced he can pull off. When he first arrived at West back in 1991, Latham was struck by how few resources his fellow PE teachers had at hand. "And I was also struck by, frankly, how fat the kids had become." By 1995, he recalls, after-school coaches were coming to him "saying, 'Look, I can't get enough kids to make a whole team anymore.'" Later, "we all got together and started talking, and it became clear right away what the enemy was — it was video games. We decided we had to find a way to make PE compete with Nintendo."

One day Latham had a brainstorm: What if they could create a gym that was one part video parlor and one part health club? He found a 2000-square-foot building on the school lot that was going unused and got the school principal to give him and his buddies permission to rehab it, with the condition that the project would not cost the district any money. Latham raised $50,000 from a local philanthropist for material costs; the labor was donated by "my coaching buddies." To equip the gym, Latham began acquiring stationary bicycles — the fancy kind used in many expensive high-tech urban health clubs. These he had wired into big video screens. On the screens appeared a number of competitive video games — which could only be played as long as the users kept on pedaling. "What we found startled us all — kids who, if you asked them to run a mile outside, would just sort of look at you and hide, they were crazy for it. I have a kid who used to weigh 310 pounds who has already dropped 50 pounds — he laughed and sweated his way through it." By 1999 Latham had raised more than $250,000. His center, which he has dubbed Cyberobics, can now accommodate up to fifty students at a time. "It's always packed," he says. It is also attracting notice. Last year, West Middle School registered big gains on the semiannual California fitness test. Students at West Middle School were number one among schools its size in the category of aerobic capacity. "Next we've gotta get that upper body strength back up," says Latham.

Perhaps the most controversial way to use schools to prevent obesity has been undertaken not by academics and health professionals, but by parents, teachers, and school administrators, who have in recent years fought a high-stakes guerrilla war with the fast-food companies that have come to dominate the school nutrition scene. The most tense battleground is that of soft drink pouring contracts, in which high schools are paid large sums of cash in exchange for an agreement to sell only one kind of soda, usually Pepsi or Coke. Also called exclusivity deals, these contracts can run into the seven-figure range — a great deal of money for any chronically hard-strapped school system. Nationally, there are thousands of such deals in place. They have, in fact, become the norm in most large school districts, with principals — and parents and administrators — justifying the consequent omnipresence of soda (and soda ads) on campus as a way to pay for athletic uniforms and a variety of after-school programs.

Such was the initial justification of most members of the Sacramento school board last year when they considered a lucrative pouring contract from Pepsi. Over a five-year period, the soft drink behemoth promised to pay the board $2.5 million in return for the exclusive right to sell and advertise Pepsi products on Sacramento public school campuses. "Frankly, it was such a done deal that when it came before us, it was expected to be fast-tracked to approval," recalls Michelle Masoner, a thirteen-year veteran of the school board. But then, after reflection, "it did not feel right to me. After all, we already had some vending machines on campuses, and many parents, and myself as a parent with kids in the district, had always felt conflicted about that. I came to believe that this contract would hook us into something long-term that we should not be selling." An associate on the board, Manny Hernandez, soon came to feel the same way. "We looked closely at the contract and saw that we were locking the kids into a long-term cycle that would be skewed to the worst nutritional situation rather than the best."

But first Masoner and Hernandez had to convince their fellow board members, who were not wont to give up the $2.5 million in free operating funds. "We decided that we had to make the health case, in very clear terms," Masoner says. At the next board meeting, her fellows heard testimony from the county coroner, who noted that arterial streaking and early signs of bone disease were being seen in children as young as ten years old. The head of the regional dental association presented epidemiological data indicating that, as he put it, "our area has the worst dental health record in the state." At the next meeting, the board unanimously rejected Pepsi's offer.

But the board did not stop there. The inquiry into the pouring contract had made them curious. And concerned. They decided to look into just how much junk food was present on campus. "What we found was stunning," Masoner says. "Candy and pop were everywhere. In almost any classroom in the district, you could find kids with soda and candy at their desk. Teachers were actually using them as a reward." Presenting all of this at a subsequent meeting, the board voted to present its principals with an ultimatum: They would have ten years to eliminate all high-sugar and high-fat foods from their campuses. The initial reaction was predictably truculent, but, say Masoner and Hernandez, the principals have more than risen to the occasion. By the end of winter break, they had already met the board's first incremental mandate of providing as much bottled water on campus as soda. "The kids were telling us they loved it," says Hernandez.

Even when the contracts themselves go unchallenged, the pouring contract disputes are increasingly fueling a new wave of parental activism. The target is junk food advertising in schools, which in recent years has become ubiquitous. The most common comes in the form of "sponsored educational materials": nutrition curriculum by McDonald's; math lessons using Tootsie Rolls and Domino's Pizza wheel graphics; reading texts that teach first graders to start out by recognizing logos from Pizza Hut and M&Ms. There is even a nutrition guide put out by McDonald's that teaches kids with diabetes how to calculate the number of diabetic "points" (the system advocated by the American Diabetes Association) in a typical McDonald's meal.

In an era when many school districts can't keep up with demand for basic texts, free supplemental materials are hard to turn away. But that is increasingly what is happening, says Andrew Hagelshaw, head of Berkeley's Center for Commercial-Free Public Education. "We are seeing hundreds of groups across the country take this issue on," he says. "The key is the parents. It's like a sleeping giant has been roused. Once they find out this has been happening right under their noses, they are unstoppable. They don't buy the notion that school is about educating consumers. It isn't. It's about educating citizens."

What can be done on a national level? Certainly obesity, with its $100 billion a year (and growing) price tag in health services, justifies some involvement by the government, or at least by large national organizations. Concern about it is now well established. On the day after the September 11, 2001, attacks, one of the few nonwar stories to break through was one about the latest obesity statistics (the national rate had jumped again — to 26 percent). A few weeks later, the army released its latest fitness study, with its own alarming obesity numbers. How can America capitalize on this growing awareness?

One way might involve expanded federal funding for safe public playgrounds and parks. There is a broad and potent constituency for such a measure, given that half of the nation's parents believe that their neighborhoods are not safe enough to let their children go outside and play. There is also the issue of pure economic equity. Recent studies in California and other states show that park and playground development has taken place disproportionately in new suburban areas, often at the expense of older — and poorer — urban centers. These same urban areas are increasingly the address of new immigrant communities who have yet to flex their political muscle on the most basic of health issues. What is needed is a revival of two older organizations, one governmental, the other private. The former would involve reinvigorating VISTA, an effective, if chronically underfunded, program that helped millions of urban Americans win basic housing and health benefits. During the 1970s and early 1980s, VISTA trained young college students to go out to poor communities and to teach residents how to organize themselves around such core issues. Another tack would focus on reviving the organizing groups of the Community Areas Foundation (CAF). Founded in the 1930s by the social activist Saul Alinsky, the CAF has successfully trained generations of urban activists on the fundamentals of how to empower local groups of citizens to demand what is their due. In the past, such groups have forced school boards to open more schools in underserved areas, pushed insurance companies to discontinue the practice of redlining, and turned back attempts to locate incinerators and toxic waste dumps in poor communities. Unfortunately, in recent years, many of the CAF groups have become bogged down in the ideological and personal antagonisms of the self-proclaimed "progressive" left. Their effectiveness has been muted, and will likely remain so until that old left dies and is replaced by a younger, more pragmatic leadership.

In California and around the nation, a perfect opportunity exists for such organizations to move the public fitness agenda forward. This is because almost every urban school district is, to one degree or another, out of compliance with state rules mandating minimal hours of physical education. California requires elementary schools to provide 100 minutes of physical education every two weeks. But few schools even come close to meeting the requirement, instead relying on recess and "unstructured playtime" to fulfill their obligations. In middle and high schools, required to provide 400 minutes every two weeks, the situation is even grimmer; studies have shown that as little as 20 percent of PE time is actually spent "in motion," the rest taken up with administrative work, suiting up, showering, and getting dressed for the next class. As one might expect, the situation degrades as the overall school performance degrades. Attempts to reduce class size in academic courses often translate into increases in PE class size. Average PE class size in Los Angeles stands at 55, with some schools logging as many as 85 kids per class. The recommended class size is 25. As the head of the Amateur Athletic Union of Los Angeles put it recently, "Someone needs to make parents aware that their children are not getting what they are entitled to, and to teach these parents how to get in the school board's face and demand what is theirs."

There is also what might be called the Americorps option. The federal program funnels newly minted college graduates into teaching and public service, providing a small but valuable support system for public schools. Yet almost all of its efforts have centered on aiding schools in the traditional academic areas graded on the SAT-9 examinations, the series of academic tests that have become the holy grail of most systems. What if it were expanded to target physical education and physical activity training? And what if the SAT-9 were broadened to include some form of fitness testing? This might seem a bit impractical, given the difficulties of so many districts in showing any progress with the most basic academic testing. A growing body of scientific and educational research, however, is documenting the connection between physical activity and mental acuity. And new studies are also documenting another link. The best academic scores among all high schools invariably match up with those displaying the best fitness scores.

We might also recast our traditional notions about food and exercise as separate pursuits toward the goal of good health. Instead, "we might start thinking of them as unified with one another," says Walter Willett, head of the Department of Nutrition at Harvard's School of Public Policy. Toward that end, Willett — the scholar who fought the USDA's ill-founded 1990 weight guidelines — has come up with an alternative food pyramid. Its principal distinction is that it defines weight control and exercise *as the base* of the pyramid. Without them — as uncomfortable as that might make parents, school administrators, and health professionals — all the healthy eating advice in the world will likely count for little, at least when it comes to obesity and the chronic disease it spawns. "And when I say exercise," adds Willett, "I mean *vigorous* exercise — enough to make you sweat!"

Then there are the "meta" approaches. Of these, the most controversial is the "fat tax." Put forth in 2000 by Yale's Kelly Brownell and Michael Jacobson at the Center for Science in the Public Interest, the proposal calls for state governments to enact small taxes on foods that are nutritionally unsound. The money would then be put into funds dedicated to promoting healthy eating and sound food choices. Despite the fact that the soft drink industry alone spends upward of $600 million annually to promote its trash (compared with the National Cancer Institute's paltry $1 million budget for promoting fruit and vegetable consumption), such promotional campaigns can be highly effective. A TV and radio campaign in Clarksburg, West Virginia, for example, encouraged shoppers to switch from higher-fat to lower-fat milk; after seven weeks, the market share for 1 percent and fat-free milk jumped from 18 to 41 percent — a change that Brownell and Jacobson note was sustained for more than a year.

But the trend in most state capitals, increasingly beholden to special interests, has been in exactly the opposite direction. There, soda and snack food lobbyists have made the elimination of such taxes a priority. In 1993 the ever-up-for-sale Louisiana legislature halved its existing soft drink tax in return for Coca-Cola's pledge to build a new bottling plant, then repealed it entirely in return for Coke building a bigger plant. At about the same time in Maryland, legislators caved in to threats from the Frito-Lay corporation not to erect a new plant there and repealed the state's snack food tax. The same story has been played out in ten other localities. If anything, these reversals serve notice to parents that the snack food industry will stoop to anything to protect its interests in maintaining their child's expanding belly, despite the medical consequences.

One might reasonably wonder, however, if the food industry might not take it upon itself to do something. It could re-size its portions. This would not require any major re-engineering for most of them. Many large snack food makers already have small-size lines in production, most of which are designed for the European market, where six to eight ounces of a soft drink have long been deemed sufficient as a portion (amusing as it may be to supersize-inclined American tourists). In recent years there has even been active consideration of introducing Euro-sizing into the United States. "But it is always held up by the basic marketing and market share imperative," says John Peters, a longtime obesity scholar who knows the food industry from the inside out. "The major players all know what could be done. But no one — no one — is going to take the first step. No one wants to take the big hit that the first to break ranks will inevitably take. They all know that, by and large, consumers are still stuck with nineteenth-century notions of 'more for less is better' in their heads."

One group of Americans has always known better than that. They are the rich, the more insightful and longer-living of whom have understood that the price of abundance is restraint; in their parlance, you can never be too rich or too thin. Yet today almost everyone in America is too rich in the fundamentals: Almost everyone has access to maximal cheap calories, and almost everyone has the opportunity to expend minimal calories. Such is the gift — and the challenge — of global capitalism, the principal legacy of Earl Butz and his war on inflation. That challenge may be one of the most difficult that modern society has ever faced. After all, overconsumption is an intuitive, rational act — at least on its face. Who wants higher food prices? Who wants to sweat? No one. Only when Americans feel the countervailing cost of being fat in their daily lives will they begin to undertake the necessary counterintuitive steps out of the obesity epidemic.

When that happens, watch out. For we need only look to previous eras to see what Americans are capable of when it comes to getting fit. In the late nineteenth century, social reformers in the mold of Jane Addams and Jacob Riis launched the playground movement, which drove hundreds of American cities to build safe, public recreation areas. Just before, German American immigrants proved extremely successful in planting a social institution known as the turnverein, or gym club, in many American communities. Often clustered around a hall and field, the turnvereins organized community members to meet on designated days of the week to exercise, dance, learn gymnastics, and practice a variety of other types of physical activity. At its peak, the movement reached far beyond its German immigrant origins to embrace a wide spectrum of the community. Before its demise in the 1920s and 1930s, due to assimilation, the turnverein had come to articulate a distinctly American view of fitness and citizenship. As one of its founders, Dr. Charles Beck, would write, there were great advantages to be derived by a republic from gymnastic exercises, "uniting in one occupation all the different classes of people and thus forming a new tie for those who, for the most part, are widely separated by their different education and pursuits of life."

There are already small — very small — signs that the nation's informal, experimental impulse is creating a new version of the public turnverein. By that I refer to the changing mode of the American Youth Soccer Organization. Until the last decade, the AYSO was largely a white, suburban phenomenon. But beginning in the early 1990s, the organization turned its efforts to cities, home to the country's burgeoning immigrant populations. The result has been an explosion of new members, and, as a result, a deeper penetration of the sport into the community. I need only spend a Friday evening on the practice field of my local middle school to witness this new phenomenon. All around the field, while boys and girls are running drills under the supervision of coaches, their waiting families are also at play. Papa teaches tiny Miguel how to skip rope. Mama jogs on the adjacent track. Brother José shoots hoops with a school friend over on the basketball court. The scene is re-created daily at hundreds of locations around the country. Instructively, all of this ancillary physical culture comes spontaneously. It is not the work of policy makers or recreation specialists but rather an expression of what happens when Americans take the time to *move*. My hope is that a variety of such responses might eventually become anchors for small but strategic new municipal investments in public fitness.

Until then, it pays to remember, perhaps while ordering that next supersized meal, that Dante put the gluttonous in the third circle of hell, where they were to endure "eternal, cold and cursed heavy rain." The slothful, one might consider as one cues up one's satellite dish, fared even worse; in the fifth circle they would "languish in the black slime" of the river Styx.

In the twenty-first century, we have put ourselves in the first circle of fat hell.

How we get out of that hell depends not upon prayer, but rather upon a new sense of collective will — and individual willpower.

Appendix:
Fat Land Facts

Notes

Index

With more food choices than ever . . .

DIETARY DIVERSITY

The number of food products introduced into the U.S. food market classified as condiments, candy, snacks, and bakery foods parallels the increasing prevalence of obesity — expressed here as body mass index (BMI) — and has increased strikingly out of proportion to new vegetable and fruit products. BMI is a health-based measure of weight for height.

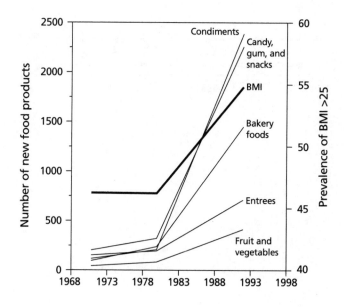

Adapted with permission from the *American Journal of Clinical Nutrition.* © *American Journal of Clinical Nutrition.* American Society for Clinical Nutrition.

. . . Americans are eating out more often . . .

**PROPORTION OF TOTAL CALORIES OBTAINED AWAY
FROM HOME ON THE RISE, 1977–1995**

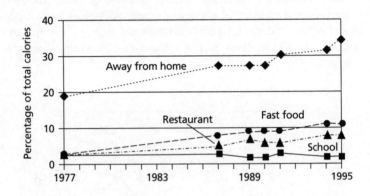

. . . eating higher-calorie meals in the process . . .

**HOME FOODS HAVE LOWER SATURATED-FAT DENSITY
THAN AWAY-FROM-HOME FOODS, 1987–1995**

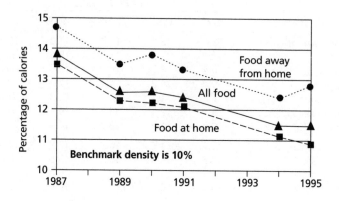

Courtesy of United States Department of Agriculture.

. . . and getting fatter by the year.

PREVALENCE OF OBESITY AMONG U.S. ADULTS, BY REGION AND STATE (Adults whose BMI [body mass index] is over 30)

REGION/STATE	PERCENT OBESE				
	1991	1995	1998	1999	2000
New England	**9.9**	**12.1**	**14.4**	**14.9**	**16.95**
Maine	12.1	13.7	17.0	18.9	19.7
New Hampshire	10.4	14.7	14.7	13.8	17.1
Vermont	10.0	14.2	14.4	17.2	17.7
Massachusetts	8.8	11.1	13.8	14.3	16.4
Rhode Island	9.1	12.9	16.2	16.1	16.8
Connecticut	10.9	11.9	14.7	14.5	16.9
Mid-Atlantic	**12.7**	**14.4**	**16.7**	**17.8**	**18.41**
New York	12.8	13.3	15.9	16.9	17.2
New Jersey	9.7	14.2	15.2	16.8	17.6
Pennsylvania	14.4	16.1	19.0	19.9	20.7
East North Central	**14.1**	**17.2**	**19.1**	**20.3**	**21.0**
Ohio	14.9	17.2	19.5	19.8	21.0
Indiana	14.8	19.6	19.5	19.4	21.3
Illinois	12.7	16.4	17.9	20.2	20.9
Michigan	15.2	17.7	20.7	22.1	21.8
Wisconsin	12.7	15.3	17.9	19.3	19.4
West North Central	**12.2**	**16.5**	**18.0**	**19.0**	**19.82**
Kansas	n/a	15.8	17.3	18.5	20.1
Minnesota	10.6	15.0	15.7	15.0	16.8
Iowa	14.4	17.2	19.3	20.9	20.8
Missouri	12.0	18.0	19.8	20.8	21.6
North Dakota	12.9	15.6	18.7	21.2	19.8
South Dakota	12.8	13.6	15.4	19.0	19.2
Nebraska	12.5	15.7	17.5	20.2	20.6
South Atlantic	**11.1**	**15.6**	**18.6**	**19.3**	**19.52**
District of Columbia	15.2	n/a	19.9	17.9	21.2
Delaware	14.9	16.2	16.6	17.1	16.2
Maryland	11.2	15.8	19.8	17.6	19.5
Virginia	10.1	15.2	18.2	18.6	17.5
West Virginia	15.2	17.8	22.9	23.9	22.8
North Carolina	13.0	16.5	19.0	21.0	21.3

REGION/STATE	PERCENT OBESE				
	1991	1995	1998	1999	2000
South Atlantic (cont.)					
South Carolina	13.8	16.1	20.2	20.2	21.5
Georgia	9.2	12.6	18.7	20.7	20.9
Florida	10.1	16.5	17.4	17.9	18.1
East South Central	**13.1**	**17.8**	**20.0**	**21.2**	**23.05**
Kentucky	12.7	16.6	19.9	21.1	22.3
Tennessee	12.1	18.0	18.5	20.1	22.7
Alabama	13.2	18.3	20.7	21.8	23.5
Mississippi	15.7	18.6	22.0	22.8	24.3
West South Central	**13.1**	**15.2**	**19.9**	**21.0**	**22.2**
Arkansas	12.7	17.3	19.2	21.9	22.6
Louisiana	15.7	17.4	21.3	21.5	22.8
Oklahoma	11.9	13.0	18.7	20.2	19.0
Texas	12.7	15.0	19.9	21.1	22.7
Mountain	**9.6**	**12.0**	**14.1**	**14.5**	**17.1**
Montana	9.5	12.6	14.7	14.7	15.2
Idaho	11.7	13.8	16.0	19.5	18.4
Colorado	8.4	10.0	14.0	14.3	13.8
New Mexico	7.8	12.7	14.7	17.3	18.8
Arizona	11.0	12.8	12.7	11.6	18.8
Wyoming	n/a	13.9	14.5	16.4	17.6
Utah	9.7	12.6	15.3	16.3	18.5
Pacific	**10.2**	**14.2**	**17.0**	**18.1**	**19.1**
Washington	9.9	13.5	17.6	17.7	18.5
Nevada	n/a	13.3	13.4	15.3	17.2
Oregon	11.2	14.7	17.8	19.6	21.0
California	10.0	14.4	16.8	19.6	19.2
Alaska	13.1	19.2	20.7	19.2	20.5
Hawaii	10.4	10.4	15.3	15.3	15.1
U.S. Total	**12.0**	**15.3**	**17.9**	**18.9**	**19.8**

Courtesy of National Center for Chronic Disease Prevention and Health Promotion.

WHAT IS YOUR BODY MASS INDEX (BMI)?

$$BMI = \frac{\text{Weight (pounds)}}{\text{Height (inches)}^2} \times 703$$

Weight in pounds

Height	120	130	140	150	160	170	180	190	200	210	220	230	240	250
4'6"	29	31	34	36	39	41	43	46	48	51	53	56	58	60
4'8"	27	29	31	34	36	38	40	43	45	47	49	52	54	56
4'10"	25	27	29	31	34	36	38	40	42	44	46	48	50	52
5'0"	23	25	27	29	31	33	35	37	39	41	43	45	47	49
5'2"	22	24	26	27	29	31	33	35	37	38	40	42	44	46
5'4"	21	22	24	26	28	29	31	33	34	36	38	40	41	43
5'6"	19	21	23	24	26	27	29	31	32	34	36	37	39	40
5'8"	18	20	21	23	24	26	27	29	30	32	34	35	37	38
5'10"	17	19	20	22	23	24	26	27	29	30	32	33	35	36
6'0"	16	18	19	20	22	23	24	26	27	28	30	31	33	34
6'2"	15	17	18	19	21	22	23	24	26	27	28	30	31	32
6'4"	15	16	17	18	20	21	22	23	24	26	27	28	29	30
6'6"	14	15	16	17	19	20	21	22	23	24	25	27	28	29
6'8"	13	14	15	17	18	19	20	21	22	23	24	25	26	28

▨ Healthy Weight　☐ Overweight　■ Obese

Note: This chart is for adults aged 20 years and older.

Courtesy of *The Surgeon General's Call to Action to Prevent and Decrease Overweight and Obesity.*

NOTES

As obesity has become linked to a growing number of chronic diseases, the number of organizations tracking it has exploded. I will note the most pertinent ones in introductory summations to chapter notes, including respective Web sites if and only if those sites provide access to primary reports and studies. The two principal journals of the field, *Obesity Research* and the *International Journal of Obesity*, both provide access to abstracts of current month contents. These are published, respectively, by the North American Association for the Study of Obesity, at www.naaso.org, and by the International Association for the Study of Obesity, at www.iaso.org. Members of both organizations have been of tremendous assistance to this work, in particular James O. Hill, of the University of Colorado Health Sciences Center.

The single most important standard work, found in all major medical libraries, is the *Handbook of Obesity*, edited by the pre-eminent George A. Bray, Claude Bouchard, and W. P. T. James (New York: Marcel Dekker, 1998). This has been joined recently by the researchers at the World Health Organization, who have produced the fine *Obesity: Preventing and Managing the Global Epidemic* (WHO Technical Report Series No. 894, 2000); some of their work can be read at www.who.int/nut/obs.htm. For another comprehensive view of obesity's health impact, see "Obesity research: a JAMA theme issue," *Journal of the American Medical Association*, v. 282, October 27, 1999; the volume has some political value as well, indicating a turn in the sentiment of a body that long viewed obesity as a legitimate medical issue with undue skepticism. Lastly there is the more recent clarion call by the U.S. surgeon general, *The Surgeon General's Call to Action to Prevent and Decrease Overweight and Obesity* (Washington,

D.C.: U.S. Department of Health and Human Services, 2001), available on
the Web at www.surgeongeneral.gov.

Introduction

3   "If obesity is left unchecked": Quoted in Associated Press, "Nearly
All Americans Will One Day Be Overweight, Researchers Predict,"
Los Angeles Times, June 29, 1998, p. A33.
"See, for decades": Interview with James Hill. For an expansion
of his views, see James O. Hill, Jeanne Goldberg, Russell Pate, and
John Peters, "Introduction to special issue," *Nutrition Reviews,* v. 59,
March 2001, pp. s4–s6 and s57–s62.

4   About 61 percent: David Satcher, Assistant Secretary for Health and
Surgeon General, *The Surgeon General's Call to Action to Prevent
and Decrease Overweight and Obesity* (Washington, D.C.: U.S. Department of Health and Human Services, 2001), p. 1. See also A. H.
Mokdad, M. K. Serdula, W. H. Dietz, *et al.,* "The spread of the obesity epidemic in the United States, 1991–1998," *Journal of the American Medical Association,* v. 282, October 27, 1999, pp. 1519–1522.
The American Bariatric Society: Quoted in Atul Gawande, "The
Man Who Couldn't Stop Eating," *The New Yorker,* July 9, 2001,
p. 78.
Children are most at risk: Overweight in childhood is reached when a
child exceeds the 85th percentile of his or her age group — that is,
when the child weighs more than 85 percent of peers; childhood obesity is reached when a child exceeds the 95th percentile. For more,
see Satcher, *Surgeon General's Call,* Figure 5, p. 5; see also *Obesity:
The Public Health Crisis* (Washington, D.C.: American Obesity Association, 1999), p. 1; note also that Richard Strauss and Harold
Pollack, "Epidemic increase in childhood overweight, 1986–1998,"
Journal of the American Medical Association, v. 286, 2001, pp.
2845–2848, offer a more nuanced look at the numbers, concluding
that "by 1998, overweight prevalence increased to 21.5 percent of African-Americans, 21.8 percent among Hispanics, and 12.3 percent
among non-Hispanic whites."
"Today," he told a group: David Satcher, Assistant Secretary for
Health and Surgeon General, "Keynote Address: USDA Conference
on Childhood Obesity" (Washington, D.C.: USDA Press Office, October 27, 1998).

5   "The lower rates": Deborah Galuska, Julie Will, Mary Serdula, and

Earl Ford, "Are health care professionals advising obese patients to lose weight?" *Journal of the American Medical Association*, v. 282, 1999, p. 157.

1. Up Up Up! (Or, Where the Calories Came From)

Despite the fact that the Nixon-Ford years provided the framework for much of what we now take for granted as "globalism," "free trade," and "open markets," no single work by a major historian has yet plumbed the political economics of that decade. Two recent books, however, treat 1970s generational politics, David Frum's *How We Got There* (New York: Perseus, 2000) and Bruce J. Schulman's *The Seventies* (New York: Free Press, 2001). The former is the livelier, conservative take, the latter being a more scholarly, liberal assessment. Both are worth reading. There is virtually no published scholarship on Earl Butz, who, at ninety-three, was gracious enough to grant me an extended phone interview from his residence in West Lafayette, Indiana. The former secretary still maintains an ambitious speaking schedule, as well as an office at Purdue University's Department of Agricultural Economics. The same university's archives were helpful in providing me access to the Butz papers, as was the staff of the Gerald R. Ford Library, in Ann Arbor, Michigan. Correspondence with Arnold Gavin, who established the first modern palm oil factories in Malaysia, was vital to understanding the origins of food oil technology. John DeCourcy, a deputy in Butz's department in the mid-1970s, was a font of detail and wisdom about the man and his politics.

7 In Washington, Butz was an optimist: Interview with John DeCourcy. Also see Julius Duscha, "Up, Up, Up — Butz Makes Hay Down on the Farm," *New York Times Magazine*, April 16, 1972, p. 73; Lillian Price, "Earl Butz — Educator, Public Servant, and the Farmer's Friend," *Lafayette Leader*, November 14, 1997, p. 4. For an example of Butz's patriotic and religious rhetoric, see Earl Butz, "Who Will Speak for America?: A Nation Under God," address, Polish Legion Veterans' Convention, August 24, 1974, in *Vital Speeches*," v. 40, September 14, 1974, pp. 710–712.

There were his endless battles with Henry Kissinger: Interview with Earl Butz. For a full explication of the USDA–State Department antagonisms, see "Memorandum for Jerry Jones," *Cabinet Meeting, October 30, 1974*, Box 3, James E. Conner Files, Gerald R. Ford Library.

7 There was his constant . . . denigration of welfare: See Duscha, "Up, Up, Up . . . ," *New York Times Magazine,* p. 90. See also "Cabinet Meeting Notes," *Cabinet Meeting, August 26, 1974,* Box 3, Conner Files.

8 "That's what it was like trying to multiply the farm vote for Nixon!": Quoted in Duscha, "Up, Up, Up . . . ," *New York Times Magazine,* p. 91.

Cautious growers simply had not planted enough grain crops: For a full account of the 1972–1973 food shortages, see "Why a Food Scare in a Land of Plenty?" *U.S. News & World Report,* v. 75, July 16, 1973, pp. 15–20.

9 By early 1973, with food price inflation at an all-time high: See chart, "As Food Supplies Dwindle . . . Prices Go Soaring," *U.S. News,* v. 75, July 16, 1973, p. 16. See also "A Threat of Food Shortage," *Time,* July 9, 1973, p. 55.

The movement even had its own graphics: "The Great Meat Furor," *Newsweek,* v. 81, April 9, 1973, p. 19.

In San Francisco . . . In Houston: *Ibid.* Also see "A Buyers' Strike That Is Succeeding," *U.S. News,* April 8, 1974, p. 20.

"Like it or not . . .": Lester R. Brown, "We Run the Risk of Empty Meat Counters," *Newsweek,* v. 75, July 16, 1973, p. 18.

10 "The only one thing in the middle of the road . . .": Quoted in Price, "Earl Butz . . . ," *Lafayette Leader,* p. 4.

To do so he launched an aggressive campaign: Earl Butz, "A Realistic Look at Food Reserves," address, December 11, 1973, in *Vital Speeches,* v. 40, January 15, 1974, pp. 197–199; Earl Butz, "Trade and Food Security," address, September 4, 1974, in *Vital Speeches,* v. 40, October 1, 1974, pp. 742–745; Earl R. Butz, "Meat Prices," address, June 29, 1972, in *Vital Speeches,* v. 38, August 15, 1972, pp. 647–649; Earl Butz, "Food, Farm Programs, and the Future," address, April 3, 1973, in *Vital Speeches,* v. 39, May 15, 1973, pp. 465–467; and Earl Butz, "Who Will Speak for America?" *Vital Speeches,* v. 40, p. 711.

For years, sugar prices: Interview, Stanley Segall, Drexel University professor of food technology. Segall is the foremost expert in the United States on added sweeteners in food processing. An outstanding overview of the need for alternatives to sugar can be found in L. Mark Hanover and John S. White, "Manufacturing, composition, and applications of fructose," *American Journal of Clinical Nutrition,* v. 58 (supp.), pp. s724–s732. See also John Long, Chapter 13, in *Alternative Sweeteners,* ed. Lyn O'Brien Nabors (New York: Marcel Dekker, 2001).

10 But in 1971 food scientists in Japan: Hanover and White, "Manufacturing . . . ," p. 724s; Y. Takasaki and Y. Kosugi, *Fermentation Advances* (New York: Academic Press, 1969); S. Akabori, K. Nehara, and I. Muramatsu, in *Journal of the Chemical Society of Japan,* v. 73, 1952, p. 311.

11 "I remember being told . . .": Segall interview. For production history of commercial fructose, see S. Vuilleumer, "Worldwide production of high-fructose syrup and crystalline fructose," *American Journal of Clinical Nutrition,* v. 58 (supp.), November 1993, pp. s733–s736.

12 Convenience foods and TV dinners . . . a ". . . maid service": Duscha, "Up, Up, Up . . . ," *New York Times Magazine,* p. 88.

A cartoon: *Ibid.*

he liked to refer to the problem as "public enemy number one": In "Cabinet Meeting Notes," *Cabinet Meeting, August 26, 1974,* Box 3.

Butz got a phone call from . . . Poage: DeCourcy interview.

13 if we were going to allow this "rat oil": DeCourcy interview; Butz interview. The entire palm oil debate is thoroughly reported, complete with Poage's remarks about "rat oil," in *Hearings Before the Subcommittee on Oilseeds and Rice and the Subcommittee on Cotton,* Committee on Agriculture, U.S. House of Representatives, Ninety-fourth Congress, Second Session, March 18, 1976; May 15, 1976; and August 5, 1976.

"It was back to square one . . .": Butz interview.

14 The stall thus lodged: DeCourcy interview. For details of Butz's "stall" as it appeared to one committee witness, see "Statement of Joe Rankin, Vice President, Texas Farmers' Union," *Hearings . . . ,* May 15, 1976, p. 141.

Palm oil had been around: A fine modern history of palm oil can be found in *Designer Oil Crops,* ed. Denis J. Murphy (Weinheim, Germany: VCH Publishing, 1994), pp. 22–27; palm oil's political and economic history is traced in James Pletcher, "Regulation with growth: the political economy of palm oil in Malaysia," *World Development,* v. 19, no. 6, 1991, pp. 623–636. For a personal account of how palm oil was refined and made commercially viable, see Arnold Gavin, "Spurring Innovations in a Fifty-Year Career," in *Scientia Gras: A Select History of Fat Science and Technology* (Champaign, Illinois: AOCS Press, 2000), pp. 73–82.

15 "Palm oil is more highly saturated than hog lard": *Hearings . . . ,* August 5, 1976, p. 75.

16 In Malaysia . . . Musa bin Hitam . . . : DeCourcy interview.

"You must realize . . .": *Ibid.* See also David A. Andelman, "Business in Malaysia," *New York Times,* August 6, 1976, p. D1.

17 "And he managed to get Hitam . . .": DeCourcy interview. Also, "Visit of H. E. Earl Butz, Secretary of Agriculture, U.S.A. and Delegation to Malaysia on 23rd April, [19]76," *Programme,* Friday, April 23; typescript memo, "Malaysia Mission," Butz Papers, Purdue University.

To Hitam he wrote . . . To DeCourcy he wrote . . . : Earl Butz, "Letter to The Honorable YB Musa bin Hitam," April 26, 1976; Earl Butz, "Letter to Mr. and Mrs. John DeCourcy, Agricultural Attaché," April 24, 1976, Butz Papers.

His most infamous — and last — official transgression: There are a number of essays and personal observations on the Butz gaffe. Two good reportorial summaries are "Butz: A Tongue Out of Order," *Newsweek,* October 11, 1976, p. 27; "The Butz Affair: He Had to Pay the Price," *U.S. News & World Report,* October 18, 1976, p. 18.

18 Prices on just about every single commodity: Darius Lakdawalla and Tomas Philipson, "The Growth of Obesity and Technological Change: A Theoretical and Empirical Examination," joint paper, presented to the American Enterprise Institute, October 18, 2001. See chart, "Changes in the Relative Price of Food in the U.S., 1951–2000," p. 3.

In what would prove to be one of the single most: See "Coke Strikes Back," *Fortune,* June 1, 1981, p. 34; Katherine Isaac, "Tate & Lyle: The Granddaddy of Sugar," *Multinational Monitor,* April 1, 1989, p. 22; Coca-Cola USA, *Annual Report,* 1980, pp. 7–9; Coca-Cola USA, *Annual Report,* 1985, p. 33.

McDonald's, which . . . fried its potatoes in palm oil: Interview and correspondence with Arnold Gavin. Between 1963 and 1984 Gavin was chief technology executive with Engineering Management Inc., a leading developer of fat- and oil-processing equipment based in Des Plaines, Illinois. It was Gavin who, while stationed in Kuala Lumpur, oversaw the development and deployment of new palm oil fractionating devices in the mid-1980s.

2. Supersize Me (Who Got the Calories into Our Bellies)

Although a number of books examine the business practices of fast-food companies — the most recent being Eric Schlosser's best-selling *Fast Food Nation* (Boston: Houghton Mifflin, 2001) — none treat the practice of supersizing in depth. Ray Kroc's *Grinding It Out: The Making of McDonald's* (Chicago: Contemporary Books, 1977) provides an entertaining inside look at the company's early years. John F. Love's *McDonald's: Behind the Arches* (New York: Bantam, 1986) was an invaluable source of journalistic leads; it also provided a basis for my examination of David Wallerstein's role in the creation of large-size fries. A boosterish but nicely reported and written look at the trade by the trade is Charles Bernstein and Ron Paul's *Winning the Chain Restaurant Game* (New York: John Wiley, 1994). A number of leads from Mr. Bernstein, the pre-eminent chronicler of the business, paid off handsomely in interviews with key industry executives. Among them were Max Cooper, a McDonald's PR executive in the 1960s, now a franchisee in Birmingham, Alabama; John Martin, the creator of the value meal concept, now an independent businessman in Irvine, California; Bob Keyser, a longtime McDonald's executive, and Bob Charles, the onetime head of the McDonald's Franchisee Advertising Association, who gave invaluable accounts of the "franchisees' revolt"; and Nancy Izquierdo, currently in the McDonald's media department, who was helpful — until her superiors curtailed all communication with me. Joanne Jacobs, corporate communications manager for McDonald's, provided general information about the company's marketing goals. Dick Forst, former head of the Burger King Franchisee Association, gave insight into that organization's concerns. Three industry trade publications, *Nation's Restaurant News, Brandweek,* and *Advertising Age,* were indispensable for establishing chronology.

20 Wallerstein had first waged war: John F. Love, *McDonald's: Behind the Arches* (New York: Bantam, 1986), pp. 296–297; Max Cooper interview; Ray Kroc, *Grinding It Out: The Making of McDonald's* (Chicago: Contemporary Books, 1977), p. 173.

21 "If people want more fries . . .": Love, *Behind the Arches,* p. 296.

22 Max Cooper, a Birmingham franchisee: Bob Keyser interview; Cooper interview; Love, *Behind the Arches,* pp. 206, 221, 224, 242, 243, 246.

23 "And we realized we could do one of three things . . .": Cooper interview.

24 In 1983 the Pepsi Corporation was looking: Teresa Carson, "Taco Bell Wants to Take a Bite Out of Burgers," *BusinessWeek,* August 4, 1986, p. 63.

"Labor, schmabor!": Quoted in Rich Karlgaard, "Interview with Susan Cramm and John Martin," *Forbes ASAP,* v. 154, August 29, 1994, p. s67.

"We had always viewed ourselves . . .": John Martin interview. See also Karlgaard, "Interview . . . ," *Forbes ASAP,* for a retrospective look at the period's innovations, as well as Bernstein and Paul's *Winning the Chain Restaurant Game.*

27 And the value meal was spreading: Brian Moran and Scott Hume, "Bigger Whopper Lets BK Throw Its Weight Around," *Advertising Age,* May 13, 1985, p. 2; Rick Van Warner, "Pizza Chains Go Head-to-Head with Two-for-One Promotions," *Nation's Restaurant News,* v. 21, July 13, 1987, p. 10.

"McDonald's must bite the bullet": Quoted in Peter O. Keegan, "McDonald's to Join 'Value' Stampede," *Nation's Restaurant News,* v. 24, December 17, 1990, p. 1; Keyser interview.

Two weeks later the front page of the same: Richard Martin, "McDonald's Kicks Off Value Menu Mix," *Nation's Restaurant News,* December 7, 1991, p. 3. For examples of how value meals and supersizing were approached by the company in later years, see "McDonald's Cuts Prices in Value Menu Move," *Marketing News,* April 1, 1991, p. 2; "War Clouds: McD, BK Arm for 79-Cent Summer Price-letting," *Brandweek,* v. 36, May 1, 1995, p. 1; and "McDonald's to Feed Value-Price Move with $66 Million in Ads," *Advertising Age,* March 3, 1997, p. 36.

A 2001 study by: Erin Lynn Morris, Elizabeth A. Bell, Liane S. Roe, and Barbara J. Rolls, "Portion size of food influences energy intake in adults," *FASEB Journal,* v. 15, March 8, 2001, p. A890.

28 Certainly the best nutritional data suggest so as well: Judy Putnam and Shirley Gerrior, "Trends in the U.S. Food Supply, 1970–1997," Chapter 7 in USDA/ERS (Economic Research Service) document AIB-750, pp. 133–160.

As of 1996 some 25 percent: Bruce Horovitz, "Portion Sizes and Fat Content Out of Control," *USA Today,* February 20, 1996. p. 1.

A serving of McDonald's french fries: See Center for Science in the Public Interest, "Monster Portions," reprinted in Jane Brody, "Fighting the Lessons Schools Teach," *New York Times,* April 16, 2002, p. D5.

By 1999 heavy users: Jennifer Ordonez, "Cash Cows: Hamburger Joints Call Them Heavy Users, but Not to Their Faces," *Wall Street Journal,* January 12, 2000, p. 1.

Twenty times a month is now McDonald's marketing goal for every: Interview with Joanne Jacobs, manager, corporate communications, McDonald's; also see Ordonez, "Cash Cows," *Wall Street Journal,* p. 1.

Little Caesar's pizza "by the foot": Bill McDowell and Laura Petrecca, "Little Caesar's Big New Idea: Pizza by the Foot," *Nation's Restaurant News,* v. 67, no. 44, 1996, p. 1.

29 "Bigness is addictive . . .": Quoted in Horovitz, "Portion Sizes . . . ,"
   USA Today, p. 1.

3. World Without Boundaries (Who Let the Calories In)

The best single source on U.S. food and nutrient consumption is the
USDA; the curious can plumb my own numbers at the agency's Web site
(www.usda.gov), which includes several recent studies on the subjects of
"away from home" dining, snacking, and overall consumption patterns.
For details about school lunch programs, I was fortunate to obtain interviews with a number of Los Angeles school nutritionists, among them
Laura Chinnock, the Los Angeles Unified School District's chief nutritionist, and Orlando Griego, then the district's director of food operations. Details of school contracts were obtained through Freedom of Information
Act requests; the major fast-food providers, Pizza Hut, Subway, and Taco
Bell, did not respond to repeated requests for interviews. A wealth of information can be found in various publications of the American School Food
Service Association, the leading professional organization for school nutritionists. I also gleaned invaluable background information from back
issues of *Food Engineering, Food Technology,* and *Quick Frozen Foods.*
Andrew Hagelshaw, the head of the Center for Commercial-Free Public
Education, was an invaluable source on the chronology of pouring and
fast-food contracts. On the subject of oversize clothing, the archives of the
Levi Strauss corporation were particularly forthcoming, as was the company's historian, Lynn Downey. The story of Big Pun was woven from a
number of personal interviews with family members and friends, to whom
I was introduced by Brian Gilmore at Loud Records; the Westchester
County Medical Examiner provided autopsy reports for the case. Interviews with Kenneth F. Ferraro, at Purdue, and R. Marie Griffith, at Prince-
ton, were indispensable in understanding the role of modern religion in
obesity.

30 "I had to wait more than an hour . . .": Charles Bernstein and Ron
   Paul, *Winning the Chain Restaurant Game* (New York: John Wiley,
   1994), pp. 63–64.
31 "We're going to go . . .": *Ibid.;* interview with Charles Bernstein.
   In 1980 even the hidebound U.S. Department of Agriculture: *The
   Hassle-Free Daily Food Guide* (Washington, D.C.: USDA, 1979).
32 The numbers show that that is exactly what the American family did:
   Biing-Hwan Lin, Joanne Guthrie, and Elizabeth Frazao, "Chapter
   12: Nutrient Contribution of Food Away from Home," in *America's*

Eating Habits: Changes and Consequences, ed. Elizabeth Frazao, Agriculture Information Bulletin 750 (Washington, D.C.: USDA, 1999), p. 213.

32 Calorically speaking, the shift: *Ibid.,* p. 217.

33 "We calculate that if food away . . .": Quoted in *Ibid.,* p. 236.
   "Where that may have been a reasonable attitude . . .": *Ibid.,* p. 237.

34 One of the more wide-ranging of these books: Harvey Diamond and Marilyn Diamond, *Fit for Life* (New York: Warner Books, 1985). "You can eat more kinds of food . . .": *Ibid.,* back cover, 1987 paperback edition.
   "Pressure causes tension": *Ibid.,* pp. 151–152.
   The authors of 1985's: Jane R. Hirschmann and Lela Zaphiropoulos, *Are You Hungry?* (New York: Random House, 1985), p. 4.
   "First, they [children] should eat . . .": *Ibid.*

35 "To questions like . . .": *Ibid.*
   As the sociologist Edward Shorter: Edward Shorter, *The Making of the Modern Family* (New York: Basic Books, 1975), p. 242; for an exception to the American rule, see "A Sample Diet for Children 7 to 12 Years," in M. V. O'Shea and John Harvey Kellogg, *Health Habits* (New York: Macmillan, 1929), pp. 122–124.

36 A counterpoint to the culture of the overfed American: For the best single treatment of the French experience, see Peter N. Stearn's excellent *Fat History* (New York: New York University Press, 1997).
   By the 1930s French medical journals were full of: See, for example, Paul Maynacher, "L'Obésité chez enfant: est elle d'origine endocrienne ou d'origine nerveuse?" (Paris: 1934).

37 "to avoid arousing his desires": Paul Strauss, *Dépopulation de Puériculture* (Paris: 1901). For the best single example of the puericulture program in action, complete with sample diets and regimens, see A. Moll-Weiss, *L'Alimentation de la Jeunesse Française* (Paris: Librarie de L'Enseignement Technique, 1931).
   And the child was never: Moll-Weiss, *L'Alimentation . . . ,* p. 31.
   "The basic message was surprisingly persistent": Stearn, *Fat History,* p. 199.

38 In a recent study by the Penn State nutrition scholar: Barbara J. Rolls, Dianne Engell, and Leann Birch, "Serving portion size influences 5-year-old but not 3-year-old children's food intakes," *Journal of the American Dietetic Association,* v. 100, February 2000, pp. 232–234.
   Far from trusting their own: *Ibid.,* p. 234.

39 Writing in the journal *Pediatrics:* H. Niinikoski, H. Lapinleimn, *et*

al., "Growth under three years of age in a prospective, randomized trial of a diet with reduced saturated fat and cholesterol," *Pediatrics,* v. 99, 1997, pp. 687–694; see also E. Obarzanek, S. Y. Kimm, B. A. Barton, L. L. Van Horn, *et al.,* "Long-term safety and efficacy of a cholesterol-lowering diet in children with elevated low-density lipoprotein cholesterol: seven-year results of the Dietary Intervention Study in Children (DISC)," *Pediatrics,* v. 107, February 2001, pp. 256–264.

39 The number and variety of high-calorie snack foods and sweets soared: Megan A. McCrory, Paul J. Fuss, *et al.,* "Dietary variety within food groups: association with energy intake and body fatness in men and women," *American Journal of Clinical Nutrition,* v. 69, 1999, pp. 440–447.

40 "Today," the Tufts researchers noted: *Ibid.*

41 To find out how much so, the pre-eminent nutrition scholar: Claire Zizza, Anna Maria-Riz, and Barry Popkin, "Significant increase in young adults' snacking between 1977–78 and 1994–96 represents a cause for concern," *Preventive Medicine,* v. 32, 2001, pp. 303–310.

"This large increase in total energy . . .": *Ibid.,* p. 303.

"Not only did hunter-gatherers . . .": Gary Frost and Anne Dornhorst, "Starting the day right way," *Lancet,* v. 357, March 10, 2001, pp. 736–737. See also Ambroise Martin *et al.,* "Is advice for breakfast consumption justified?" *British Journal of Nutrition,* v. 84, 2000, pp. 333–344.

43 The old, wide-ranging interpretation of *in loco parentis:* The classic definition can be found in Blackstone's Commentaries, Book One, Chapter 16. For a more contemporary discussion, see James Q. Wilson, "In Loco Parentis," *The Brookings Review,* Fall 1993, pp. 12–15; see also Kern Alexander and M. David Alexander, *The Law of Schools, Students and Teachers in a Nutshell* (St. Paul: West Publishing, 1984).

As Thomas R. McDaniel wrote: Thomas R. McDaniel, *The Teacher's Dilemma* (Lanham, Md.: University Press of America, 1983), p. 16.

Its principal proponent, a cigar-chomping: David Frum, *How We Got Here: The Seventies* (New York: Basic Books, 2000), pp. 325–326; Bruce J. Schulman, *The Seventies* (New York: Free Press, 2001), pp. 206–215; Joel Kotkin and Paul Grabaowitz, *California Inc.* (New York: Rawson, Wade, 1982).

44 In 1981 the California Department of Education: Interview with Laura Chinnock; interview with Gene White.

44 "What that did was to force us . . .": Chinnock interview.
45 "If the school cafeteria couldn't cook the meals . . .": White interview. For the experiences of other major cities, see David Nakamura, "Schools Hooked on Junk Food," *Washington Post,* February 27, 2001, p. A1.
46 The answer came in the early 1990s, when a group: Chinnock interview; interview with Andrew Hagelshaw.
"it was as if this huge light bulb . . .": Interview with Project Lean member, who requested anonymity. Project Lean is a statewide organization advocating major changes within the school food programs. Also, interview with Jackie Domac, nutrition instructor, Venice High School.
But the single most important innovation: "Agreement, Domino's Pizza Inc. and Los Angeles Unified School District," signed June 1, 1998, and "Agreement, Pizza Hut Inc. and Los Angeles Unified School District," signed June 1, 1998. Also Chinnock interview; White interview; interview with Orlando Griego.
47 By 1999, 95 percent of 345 California high schools: "Fact Sheet: 2000 California High School Fast Food Survey" (Berkeley: Public Health Institute, 2000).
Portion sizes for pizza were a case in point: "Product Specifications: Pizza Wedge," Item 4 A, B, from LAUSD Food Services Product Specifications; "Pizza Hut Agreement," p. 2; "Domino's Agreement," p. 3.
48 "The concern was that somehow that would affect the taste . . .": Chinnock interview.
"The response was nil . . .": *Ibid.*
This time the inducements came in the form of: "Contract, Coca-Cola Bottling and Venice High School," April 2001; also see Eric Schlosser, *Fast Food Nation* (Boston: Houghton Mifflin, 2001), pp. 51–55; Nakamura, "Schools Hooked on Junk Food"; interview with Jackie Domac.
49 Between 1989 and 1994 consumption of soft drinks: Joan F. Morton and Joanne F. Guthrie, "Changes in children's total fat intakes," *Family Economics and Nutrition Review,* v. 11, 1998, pp. 48–49; Lisa Harnack, Jamie Stang, and Mary Story, "Soft drink consumption among U.S. children and adolescents: nutritional consequences," *Journal of the American Dietetic Association,* v. 99, April 1999, pp. 436–441.
"Compensation for energy consumed in liquid . . .": David S. Ludwig, Karen E. Peterson, and Steven L. Gortmaker, "Relation between

consumption of sugar-sweetened drinks and childhood obesity," *Lancet*, v. 357, February 17, 2001, pp. 505–508.

50 The lone dissenter was a Cornell University: Robert C. Atkins, *Dr. Atkins' Diet Revolution* (New York: Bantam, 1973).

Banting, who lost some fifty pounds: William Banting, *On Corpulence* (London: Harrison and Sons, 1864), 3rd ed. See also Hillel Schwartz, *Never Satisfied* (New York: Anchor, 1986), pp. 100–101; Greg Critser, "Today's Diet Moguls Could Learn from the Victorians," *USA Today*, March 1, 2000, p. A19.

52 In 1989 W. W. Norton published: Martin Katahn, *The T-Factor Diet* (New York: W. W. Norton, 1989).

"Dr. Ornish's program . . .": Dean Ornish, *Eat More, Weigh Less* (New York: HarperCollins, 1993).

"Basta with pasta!": Barry Sears, *The Zone Diet* (New York: HarperCollins, 1995).

That same year Bantam: Michael Eades and Mary Dan Eades, *Protein Power* (New York: Bantam, 1995).

53 There had been legitimate scientific debate about: For a good overview of nineteenth-century thought on liver function, see Patricia B. Swan, "Experiments that changed nutritional thinking," paper read at Experimental Biology 95 symposium (Atlanta, Georgia), April 11, 1995. See also Claude Bernard, *An Introduction to the Study of Experimental Medicine* (New York: Dover, 1957), trans. Henry Copley Greene.

To be fair, it had never had a very bad one: Interview with R. Marie Griffith; R. Marie Griffith, "The Promised Land of Weight Loss," *Christian Century*, May 7, 1997, pp. 448–454; Solomon Schimmel, *The Seven Deadly Sins* (New York: Free Press, 1992).

The early nineteenth century's Sylvester Graham: See Steven Nissenbaum, *Sex, Diet and Debility: Sylvester Graham and Diet Reform* (Westport, Conn.: 1980), pp. 5–8. See also Schwartz, *Never Satisfied*, pp. 15–49.

54 "When God first dreamed you into creation": Griffith, "The Promised Land of Weight Loss," p. 448. Also, Charlie W. Shedd, *Pray Your Weight Away* (Philadelphia: J. B. Lippincott, 1957), pp. 15, 90–96. For a modern version of Shedd, targeted at Christian women, see Gwen Shamblin, *The Weigh Down Diet* (New York: Doubleday, 1997).

"Today my body belongs to God . . .": Shedd, *Pray Your Weight Away*, p. 90.

"he balanced his moral rebuke . . .": Griffith interview.

54 "Literalists are prone to view . . .": Chris Smith, "Fat Christians in an Age of Hunger," *Communique: A Quarterly Journal,* 1st quarter, 1999, p. 1.

55 At places like Fuller Seminary: Author interview.

The end result of this reorientation: Griffith interview.

As the sociologist Émile Durkheim: Émile Durkheim, *The Elementary Forms of the Religious Life* (London: George Allen & Unwin, 1915), pp. 47, 227, 419.

God and society "are only one": *Ibid.,* p. 206.

56 In a 1998 study looking at 3500 U.S. adults: See Kenneth F. Ferraro, "Firm believers? Religion, body weight, and well-being," *Review of Religious Research,* v. 39, March 1998, pp. 224–244.

"Consolation and comfort from religion and from eating": *Ibid.,* p. 236.

"There is no evidence of religion . . .": *Ibid.,* p. 231.

57 "They feel they would risk alienating . . .": Interview with Kenneth Ferraro. For an expansion of Ferraro's work, see Kenneth Ferraro, "Does religion influence adult health?" *Journal for the Scientific Study of Religion,* v. 30, 1991, pp. 193–202; Kenneth Ferraro and Jerome Koch, "Religion and health among black and white adults," *Journal for the Scientific Study of Religion,* v. 33, 1994, pp. 362–375; and Kenneth Ferraro and Tara Booth, "Age, body mass index, and functional illness," *Journal of Gerontology,* v. 54b, 1999, pp. s339–s348.

"I know gluttony is a bad thing . . .": Quoted in Smith, "Fat Christians in an Age of Hunger."

By the mid-1980s, however, both Levi Strauss: Interview with Lynn Downey, Historian, Levi Strauss & Co. Also "List of Sizes: 1915, Levi Strauss," "Ages and Sizes: 1920, Levi Strauss," "Ages and Sizes, 1950, Levi Strauss Catalogue," "Men's and Young Men's Sizes: 1961 Levi Strauss Catalogue," "Blue Levi's: 1970, Levi Strauss Catalogue."

58 "We about a buncha obese playboys!": Riggs Morales, "Heavyweight Champion," *The Source,* February 1999, pp. 154–158.

"A lot of Latinos and blacks are overweight . . .": Interview with "Fat Joe," Pun's recording partner and producer.

The record company that eventually: See *Loud Records Biography* (New York: Sony Music, 1999).

By 1998 Pun had ballooned: Interview with "Cuban Link," Pun's fellow band member. See also Riggs Morales and Kim Osorio, "Larger Than Life," *The Source,* May 2000, p. 183.

58 "They got him whatever he wanted": Interview with "Boovie," Pun's cousin.

59 "People would tie his shoes for him . . .": Interview with "Erica," Pun associate, anonymity requested.

By the time he was twenty-nine, when he died of a massive heart attack, he weighed 698 pounds: See Louis Roh, Medical Examiner, Westchester County, "Autopsy Report: Christopher Rios," #M2000–0335, February 8, 2000, p. 2.

60 "They were huge . . .": Interview with Johannes Hebebrand, University of Marburg.

Large sizes account for a growing: Leslie Earnest, "Plus-Size Youths Are Getting More Fashion Choices," *Los Angeles Times,* April 16, 2001, p. C1. See also Deborah Belgum, "Livin' Large," *Los Angeles Business Journal,* April 9, 2001, p. 44.

"This is one of the hot new target audiences": Quoted in Constance L. Hayes, "The Media Business: Advertising," *New York Times,* February 27, 2002, p. C10.

61 Garrow's obese patients: J. S. Garrow and G. T. Gardiner, "Maintenance of weight loss in obese patients after jaw wiring," *British Medical Journal,* v. 282, March 14, 1981, pp. 858–860.

62 About two months after: Bernstein and Paul, *Winning the Chain Restaurant Game,* p. 63.

4. Why the Calories Stayed on Our Bodies

Though America is supposedly fixated on the subject of fitness, there are few decent texts on the history of physical education in the United States. One worth reading, despite its age, is Emmett A. Rice's outstanding *A Brief History of Physical Education* (New York: A. S. Barnes, 1926). Fortunately, primary sources abound. At the National Archives in College Park, Maryland, I examined the entire documentary record of the President's Council on Physical Fitness and Sports (1956–present), which provided important analytical and narrative records of that influential body. The council's *Research Digest* was particularly helpful.

A number of leading fitness authorities granted me extensive interviews, among them the University of Arizona's Charles Corbin, who, with his associate Bob Pangrazi, may well be the most influential academic in the field of fitness today. Ash Hayes, onetime director of the president's council, also granted me several lengthy interviews. So did John Cates, who served as deputy to council presidents George Allen and Arnold

Schwarzenegger. Betty Hennessy, of the Los Angeles County Department of Education, was a font of information on the local front, where she remains a forceful proponent of public fitness. The American Alliance for Health, Physical Education, Recreation and Dance (AAHPERD) was a source of background information on the subject of fitness testing.

The Cooper Institute provided extensive information about its continuing fitness study; much of its work — and that of others involved in fitness policy — can be found in the annals of *Medicine and Science in Sports and Exercise,* the *Journal of the American Medical Association,* the *Lancet,* and *Archives of Internal Medicine.* In addition to interviews with key players such as Walter Willett, Meir Stampfer, and C. Wayne Callaway in the 1990 weight guidelines debate, I also received extensive archival transcripts from the USDA's Center for Nutrition Policy and Promotion.

63 As president of the President's Council: Interview with John Cates. See also "Youth Fitness Summits: A. Schwarzenegger," Boxes 17–20, *Papers of the President's Council on Physical Fitness,* National Archives, College Park, Maryland, hereafter abbreviated as *PPCPF.*

64 On his better days: "Meeting Minutes," May 1, 1990, Box 12, *PPCPF.*
"I just don't understand": "Meeting Minutes," September 25, 1990, Box 12, *PPCPF.*
He suspected the American Alliance . . . of: "Meeting Minutes," April 5, 1990, Box 12, *PPCPF.*
"We had thirteen lawyers . . .": Cates interview. See also "Meeting Minutes," May 1, 1990, *PPCPF.*
The last indignity came: Cates interview.

65 Nowhere was this more apparent than in California: See *Healthy Bodies, Healthy Minds: A Study of the Decline of Physical Education in California Schools* (Sacramento: Assembly Office of Research, 1984), pp. 49–51; for a national overview of PE and government until 1941, see Gwendolyn Drew, *A Historical Study of the Concern of the Federal Government for the Physical Fitness of Non-age Youth with Reference to the Schools* (Pittsburgh, Pennsylvania: Ph.D. dissertation, University of Pittsburgh, 1944).

66 To accommodate them, PE staffs were: *Healthy Bodies, Healthy Minds,* pp. 8–9, 11–14.

67 "Staffing has been reduced . . .": *Ibid.,* p. 3.
"teachers were on their own": Interview with Betty Hennessy.
By 1980 another Department of Education survey: *Healthy Bodies, Healthy Minds,* pp. 11, 18.

68 "We as physical educators . . .": Cates interview.
Overnight the new law sliced: Philip J. LaVelle, "Tax Revolt: No Minor Proposition," *San Diego Union-Tribune,* June 14, 1998, p. 1.
By 1980 average PE class sizes had doubled: *Healthy Bodies, Healthy Minds,* pp. 3, 11–23.

69 "In a time of financial strain . . .": *Ibid.,* p. 13. For a retrospective look at the impact of Proposition 13, see LaVelle, "Tax Revolt." See also Lynell George, "Testing the Teachers," *Los Angeles Times,* June 27, 1996, p. E1.
Founded at an impromptu get-together: "Twenty-fifth Anniversary Album" (Hawthorne, California: AYSO Publications, 1989), pp. 4–5.

70 "It really wasn't until later . . .": Interview with Lollie Keyes, chief communications officer, AYSO. For a full discussion of sports clubs and class, see Vern D. Seefeldt and Martha E. Ewing, "Youth sports in America," *PCPFS Research Digest,* v. 2, no. 11. In a wide-ranging statistical review of youth participation in sports clubs from 1954 to 1992, the authors concluded, "While the number of youth involved in organized sports programs is impressive, the opportunities to engage in sports programs are unequal across genders and social classes. Greater opportunities exist among children who grow up in middle and upper classes where resources enable adults to sponsor, organize, and administer programs for their children."
All of this . . . Yankelovich: Quoted in Karen Jacobs, "The Pay Gap," *Wall Street Journal,* May 1, 2000, p. R7.
they were not urbanites but rather urban villagers: For an engaging and relevant exposition of the Italian Americans corollary, see Herbert J. Gans, *The Urban Villagers* (Toronto: Free Press of Glencoe, 1962), especially pp. 45–197.

71 "always says yes": Jacobs, "The Pay Gap." See also C. O. Airhihenbuwa, S. Kumanyika, T. D. Agurs, and A. Lowe, "Perceptions and beliefs about exercise, rest, and health among African-Americans," *Annals of Internal Medicine,* v. 1, 1993: 650–654.
"has the potential to do more harm than good": Airhihenbuwa *et al.,* "Perceptions and beliefs . . . ,": p. 651.
Consider a 2000 study of 1929: *Ibid.*

72 "Adults who perceive they have too little . . .": Larry A. Tucker, "Television viewing and exercise habits of 8885 adults," *Perceptual and Motor Skills,* v. 77, 1993, p. 938.
"Children are naturally very active . . .": Quoted in E. G. A. H. van Mil, A. H. C. Goris, and K. R. Westerterp, "Physical activity and the prevention of childhood obesity," *International Journal of Obesity,* v. 23, 1999, pp. s42–s44.

72 "Kids and dads watching twenty-three . . .": Interview with Larry Tucker.

73 What was surprising, though, was the pronounced class and: Ross Andersen, Carlos Crespo, *et al.,* "Relationship of physical activity and television watching with body weight and level of fatness among children: results from the third national health and nutrition survey," *Journal of the American Medical Association,* v. 279, 1998, pp. 28–32.

About 46 percent of all U.S. adults: *Ibid.*

74 "boys and girls who watched four or more . . .": *Ibid.*

A study by the Amateur Athletic Union: Cited and graphed in R. V. Luepker, "How physically active are American children and what can we do about it?" *International Journal of Obesity,* v. 23, 1999, pp. s12–s17.

In California, the onetime model of: Duke Helfand, "State Youths Flunk Fitness Exam," *Los Angeles Times,* December 11, 2001, p. B1; Greg Critser, "A Get Fit Plan for Physical Education," *Los Angeles Times,* December 16, 2001, p. M3.

75 A growing number of Latino children were showing up: Interview with Dr. Francine Kaufman, chief, endocrinology and metabolism, director, Comprehensive Childhood Diabetes Center, Children's Hospital Los Angeles.

76 "Not only had the sport segregated itself . . .": Interview with Steve Pezman.

Fortune magazine, in a typical screed: "A Proposal for Fat City," *Fortune,* December 14, 1981, p. 4.

"All of us must consider our own responsibilities . . .": Quoted in "Fitness in Action," newsletter, March 1961, Box 1, *PPCPF.* See also John F. Kennedy, "The Vigor We Need," *Sports Illustrated,* July 16, 1962, p. 12; for an example of the Cold War context and how it shaped the early council, see Bud Wilkenson, "In a Dangerous World, Is American Youth Too Soft?" *U.S. News & World Report,* August 21, 1961, pp. 75–78.

77 There were specialized fitness magazines: *Vim: A Complete Exercise Plan for Girls 12–18,* and *Vigor: A Complete Exercise Plan for Boys 12–18,* President's Council on Physical Fitness, 1963, Box 1, *PPCPF.*

There was a council theme song: "115K Copies of 'Go You Chicken Fat Go' Sold," *Fitness News,* November 1963, Box 1, *PPCPF.*

"In 1958 the average . . .": Stan Musial, "Introduction: Closing the Muscle Gap," *Four Years for Fitness 1961–1965: A Report to the*

President (Washington, D.C.: President's Council, 1966), p. 3, Box 1, *PPCPF.*

78 "My parents had moved there": Interview with Ash Hayes.
He also assumed a headache: *National School Population Fitness Survey* (Washington, D.C.: PCPFS, 1985), pp. 23–31; Ash Hayes, "Youth physical fitness hearings," *Journal of Physical Education, Recreation and Dance,* v. 55, pp. 29–40; "Study Sparks Change in Presidential Award Program," *Newsletter: PCPFS,* May 1985, p. 1.

79 But for Hayes, that wasn't: "Two National Studies Indicate America's Young People Out of Shape," *Newsletter: PCPFS,* October 1985, p. 2.
"My total budget was $1.5 million": Hayes interview.

80 The first was the ascendance of aerobic exercise: Kenneth H. Cooper, *Aerobics* (Philadelphia: J. B. Lippincott, 1968).

81 "Basically, the same kids won it year after year": Interview with Charles Corbin.

82 As Hayes saw it: Hayes interview; "Background 2.1: Introduction," *National School Population Fitness Survey,* pp. 3–5; Ash Hayes, "Memorandum for the Record: Chronology of Events Relative to Youth Physical Fitness Testing and the Presidential Fitness Award," July 7, 1986, copy provided to author by Ash Hayes.

83 "There was a whole self-esteem issue . . .": Cates interview.
To reconcile the two tests: Hayes interview; Corbin interview; Hayes, "Memorandum . . . ," pp. 2–3.
Then, just as both groups: Corbin interview; Hayes interview; An independent narrative is found in "Meeting Minutes," April 1991, pp. 45–55, Box 13, *PPCPF.* According to testimony by Warren Giese, "The AAPHERD [*sic*] people at the final meeting sat down and . . . looked us all in the eye and said either you use the test that we scientists say is the test that is supposed to be used which included a skin fold test which this Council absolutely refused to accept and that started us off as to we would not use the test . . . the basic rupture was because AAPHERD was going to tell the President's Council either we use that test or else."
"wasn't ever in the business of making weight an issue": Hayes interview.

84 In one ad depicting: "Ad Council," Box 4, *PPCPF.* The identification and reporting of overweight and obesity were part of the original council mission, as evidenced in the 1961 guide, published by the council, entitled *Youth Physical Fitness: Suggested Elements of a School-Centered Program.* The guide states (p. 7) that "health appraisal proce-

dures should include . . . height and weight measurements, interpreted in terms of individual needs; pupils who are obviously obese, underweight or malnourished should be identified and referred to the medical authorities" (Box 1, *PPCPF*). See also "A Special Note About Weight," in Bud Wilkenson, *Official U.S. Physical Fitness Program* (Washington, D.C.: President's Council, 1962), p. 7.

84 "As we saw it . . . body fat testing . . .": Corbin interview.

85 "We were basically shut out": *Ibid.* Also interview with Dr. Judy Young, president, AAHPERD.

"15–60 minutes of continuous aerobic activity": American College of Sports Medicine, "Position Stand on the Recommended Quantity and Quality of Exercise for Developing and Maintaining Fitness in Healthy Adults," 1978. For a thorough chronological review of the standards and their weakening, see also S. N. Blair, R. S. Paffenbarger, H. W. Kohl, and N. F. Gordon, "How much physical exercise is good for health?" *Annual Review of Public Health,* v. 13, 1992, pp. 99–126.

86 "Adequate exercise means vigorous exercise": J. N. Morris, R. Pollard, *et al.,* "Vigorous exercise in leisure-time: protection against coronary heart disease," *Lancet,* December 6, 1980, pp. 1207–1210.

Experts attributed this to the modern lifestyle: Only recently have hard population data emerged on this point. An outstanding recent work looking at the period 1982–1989 showed a substantial rise in the percentage of least strenuous jobs and a substantial drop in the percentage of most strenuous jobs. See Table One in Darius Lakdawalla and Tomas Philipson, "The Growth of Obesity and Technological Change" (Santa Monica: RAND Institute, 2001).

87 On both these accounts . . . Harvard . . . Cooper's: Ralph Paffenbarger, Jr., Alvin Wing, and Robert Hyde, "Physical activity as an index of heart attack risk in college alumni," *American Journal of Epidemiology,* v. 108, September 1978, pp. 161–175; Ralph Paffenbarger, Jr., *et al.,* "The association of changes in physical-activity level and other lifestyle characteristics with different mortality among men," *New England Journal of Medicine,* v. 328, February 1993, pp. 525–545; Steven N. Blair, Harold Kohl, Ralph S. Paffenbarger, Jr., *et al.,* "Physical fitness and all-cause mortality," *Journal of the American Medical Association,* v. 262, November 1989, pp. 2395–2401.

"If there is a causal relationship": Paffenbarger, Wing, and Hyde, "Physical Activity . . . ," p. 166.

88 "High intensity exercise affords little additional benefit": Robert

DeBusk, Ulf Stenestrand, *et al.*, "Training effects of long versus short bouts of exercise in healthy subjects," *American Journal of Cardiology*, v. 65, April 1990, pp. 1010–1013.

88 "A brisk walk of 30–60 minutes . . .": Blair, Kohl, *et al.*, "Physical Fitness and . . . ," p. 2400.

The American Heart Association was the first: Gerald Fletcher, Victor Froelicher, *et al.*, "Exercise standards: a statement for health professionals from the American Heart Association," *Circulation*, v. 82, December 1990, p. 2307.

89 Even the authors of the Cooper and Harvard: Blair, Paffenbarger, *et al.*, "How much physical exercise . . . ," p. 102.

In 1993 they seized control: Centers for Disease Control, American College of Sports Medicine, President's Council on Physical Fitness, *Summary Statement: Workshop on Physical Activity and Public Health* (Indianapolis: American College of Sports Medicine, 1993).

After all, only six months before: Paffenbarger *et al.*, "The Association of Changes . . . ," p. 544.

90 "was under tremendous pressure . . .": Interview with Walter Ettinger, M.D., Wake Forest University.

91 Consider what they wrote in the aftermath: Quoted in Paul Williams, "Relationship of distance run per week to coronary heart disease risk factors in 8283 male runners," *Archives of Internal Medicine*, v. 157, January 1997, p. 191.

93 The authors, led by Stanford's Robert F. DeBusk: DeBusk, Stenestrand, *et al.*, "Training effects . . . ," p. 1010.

Peak oxygen intake: *Ibid.*

"multiple short bouts . . . as a single long bout": *Ibid.*, p. 1013.

"In contrast . . . increasing the overall daily . . .": Paul Williams, "Physical fitness and activity as separate heart disease risk factors: a meta-analysis," *Medicine and Science in Sports and Exercise*, 2001, pp. 754–761.

94 "Our data suggest that substantial health benefits . . .": Williams, "Relationship of distance . . . ," p. 191.

"Formulating physical activity recommendations . . .": Williams, "Physical Fitness and Activity . . . ," p. 754.

"overall, there is a consistent inverse dose-response": Y. Antero Kesaniemi, Elliot Danforth, Jr., *et al.*, "Dose-response issues concerning physical activity and health: an evidence-based symposium," *Medicine and Science in Sports and Exercise*, v. 33, supp., June 2001, p. s354.

95 The ACSM itself recently published: Claude Bouchard, "Physical activity and health: introduction to the dose-response symposium," *Medicine and Science in Sports and Exercise*, v. 33, supp., June 2001, p. s348.

"current strategies have not been very successful . . .": Frank B. Hu, Joanne E. Manson, "Diet, lifestyle, and the risk of type 2 diabetes mellitus in women," *New England Journal of Medicine,* v. 345, September 2001, pp. 790–797, see especially Table 1. See also F. B. Hu, R. J. Sigal, *et al.,* "Walking compared with vigorous physical activity and risk of diabetes in women: a prospective study," *Journal of the American Medical Association,* v. 282, October 1999, pp. 1433–1439; M. J. Stampfer, F. B. Hu, J. E. Manson, E. B. Rimm, and W. C. Willett, "The primary prevention of coronary heart disease in women through diet and lifestyle," *New England Journal of Medicine,* v. 343, 2000, pp. 16–22; F. B. Hu, M. J. Stampfer, J. E. Manson, G. A. Colditz, and W. C. Willett, "Trends in the incidence of coronary heart disease and changes in diet, and lifestyle, in women," *New England Journal of Medicine,* v. 343, 2000, pp. 530–537.

Noting that members of the Weight Registry: *Transcripts of Proceedings: Dietary Guidelines Advisory Committee* (Washington, D.C.: USDA), September 28, 1998, pp. 102–104.

"the assumption [is] that most people . . .": Bouchard, "Physical activity and health . . . ," p. s349.

The guidelines are promulgated every five years: Carol Davis and Etta Saltos, "Dietary Recommendations and How They Have Changed Over Time," in *America's Eating Habits* (Washington, D.C.: USDA/Economic Research Service), publication AIB-750, p. 45 for chart.

97 "At what weight-for-height ranges does minimum mortality . . .": R. Andres, D. Elahi, *et al.,* "Impact of age on weight goals," *Annals of Internal Medicine,* v. 103, 1985, pp. 1031–1033.

"the Metropolitan Life tables have erred . . .": *Ibid.,* p. 1032.

"We compared the body mass . . .": *Ibid.,* p. 1031.

98 "systematic underestimate of the impact of obesity . . .": JoAnn Manson, Meir Stampfer, Charles Hennekens, and Walter Willett, "Body weight and longevity: a reassessment," *Journal of the American Medical Association,* v. 257, 1987, pp. 353–358.

99 "few in the general U.S. population . . . excessive leanness": *Ibid.,* p. 358.

100 "I can line up ten people . . .": Interview with Wayne Callaway.

"lets men off the hook too easily": *Ibid.* See also *Transcripts of Pro-*

ceedings: Dietary Guidelines Advisory Committee, January 10, 1990, p. 212.

101 To Callaway, such a statement was "authoritarian": See also *Transcripts of Proceedings,* August 10, 1989, p. 97.

"But that concept still has to be conveyed . . .": *Ibid.,* pp. 97–98.

"Because if we look at certain subsegments . . .": *Transcripts of Proceedings,* August 5, 1989, p. 110.

"By the time a woman gets to age sixty-five . . .": *Ibid.,* p. 106.

"our views did not get a fair shake": Interview with Meir Stampfer.

102 "As far as I am concerned": Interview with Walter Willett.

As the *New York Times* put it: Denise Webb, "What Is a Healthful Diet?" *New York Times,* November 7, 1990, p. C3.

For the next five years . . . a broad swath: For an example, see "Weight, weight change, and coronary heart disease in women," *Journal of the American Heart Association,* v. 273, 1995, pp. 461–465, and citations therein.

"Based on published data, there appears to be no justification . . .": *Report of the Dietary Guidelines Advisory Committee on the Dietary Guidelines for Americans, 1995* (Washington, D.C.: Human Nutrition Information Service, USDA).

103 "Fit, fat, and bald . . .": Quoted in Linda Villarosa, "New Fatness Guidelines Spur Debate on Fitness," *New York Times,* June 23, 1998, p. F7.

He has run, by his own estimate: Laura Beil, "Fatness, Fitness Can Coexist," *Dallas Morning News,* August 30, 1999, Health Section, p. 1.

"We've got to get rid of this focus on weight": Quoted in Emma Thomas, "Study Finds Obese Exercisers Outlive Thin People Who Don't," *Tulsa World/Associated Press,* July 19, 2001.

"Let's throw away all the scales . . .": Beil, "Fatness, Fitness . . ."

"you can stay overweight and obese . . .": Thomas, "Study Finds Obese Exercisers . . ."

The test starts at a speed of eighty-eight: Carolyn Barlow, Harold Kohl, Larry Gibbons, and Steven N. Blair, "Physical fitness, mortality and obesity," *International Journal of Obesity,* v. 19, supp. 4, 1995, pp. s41–s44.

104 "inverse gradients of mortality . . . were similar for obese . . .": *Ibid.,* p. s44.

"The health benefits of normal weights appear to be limited . . .": C. D. Lee, A. S. Jackson, and S. N. Blair, "U.S. weight guidelines: is it also important to consider cardiorespiratory fitness?" *International Journal of Obesity,* v. 22, supp. 2, 1998, pp. s2–s7.

105 The media translation was predictable: Thomas, "Study Finds Obese Exercisers . . ."
A book came out that was entitled: Judy Molnar and Bob Babbitt, *You Don't Have to Be Thin to Win* (New York: Villard, 2000).
The *New York Times* even went so far: Jane E. Brody, "Fat but Fit: A Myth About Obesity Is Slowly Being Debunked," *New York Times,* October 24, 2000, p. D7.
Blair admitted: "Men with a BMI >30 . . .": Barlow, Kohl, Gibbons, and Blair, "Physical fitness, mortality . . . ," pp. s41–s42.
"The highest death rate": *Ibid.,* p. s42.
And when one looks at the *difference* between: *Ibid.,* see chart, p. s42.

106 "Men who were normal weight . . .": Lee, Jackson, and Blair, "U.S. weight guidelines: is it . . . ," p. s4.
Of Blair's total universe of people, 8100: *Ibid.,* chart, p. s5.

107 Alexander is also, at 5'8" and 260 pounds, "a big boy": Quoted in Foster Klug, "Being Fat Doesn't Mean He's Not Fit," *Sunday Washington Times*/Associated Press, February 11, 2001.
"The most important risk factor for type 2 diabetes . . .": Hu and Manson, "Diet, lifestyle, and the risk of type 2 . . . ," p. 795.
"More than 61 percent . . .": *Ibid.*
the laboratory of so-called Syndrome X: Gerald Reaven, *Syndrome X: Overcoming the Silent Killer That Can Give You a Heart Attack* (New York: Simon & Schuster, 2000), pp. 47–60.

108 A pound of extra body weight: Interview with Dr. Michael Ellman, rheumatologist, University of Chicago, quoted in Jerry Adler, "Arthritis: What It Is, Why You Get It, and How to Stop the Pain," *Newsweek,* September 3, 2001, p. 44.

5. What Fat Is, What Fat Isn't

In the popular press, the subject of class and fat has been obscured, at least for the past two decades, by identity politics. Not so in the academic press. In epidemiological literature, an abundance of data has been accumulated, and is routinely reported in the influential *Annals of Epidemiology.* So too in two professional journals, *Obesity Research* and *International Journal of Obesity,* as in the profession's bible, the *Handbook of Obesity.* A number of original works on the subject of anorexia, obesity, and eating disorders can be found on the Web sites of the Centers for Disease Control, the National Institute for Diabetes and Digestive and Kidney Disease, and the U.S. Surgeon General. On the anthropology of obesity I was fortunate to interview Deborah Crooks at the University of Kentucky at Lexington. On the subject of body image and body weight testing, James Whitehead at the University of North Dakota was of particular help. About the fat rights movement, Michael Fumento has written an engaging and informative book on the subject, *The Fat of the Land* (New York: Viking Penguin, 1997), well worth your time.

110 At the very bottom end were households: See the chart in David Barboza, "Rampant Obesity, a Debilitating Reality for the Urban Poor," *New York Times,* December 26, 2000, p. D5.

"The relationship of income and obesity . . .": Sue Y. Kimm, Eva Obarzanek, *et al.,* "Race, socioeconomic status, and obesity in 9- to 10-year-old girls: the NHLBI growth and health study," *Annals of Epidemiology,* v. 6, 1996, pp. 272–273.

111 There, obesity has become the defining . . . : Stephanie Mencimer, "Hiding in Plain Sight," *Washington City Paper,* June 16, 2000, pp. 22–32.

112 "The adolescents . . .": *Ibid.,* pp. 23–24.

"It's tiresome . . .": *Ibid.,* p. 24; for a summary of research on poverty's impact on one's ability to solve life's problems, see also Faith McLellan, "Countering poverty's hindrance of neurodevelopment," *Lancet,* v. 359, 2002, p. 236.

Much of that cocoon: Michael Stamler, "SBA Loan Guarantees, Select Cities, 1982–2001," *Report in Response to Memo from Greg Critser,* Small Business Administration, February 21, 2001; Eric Schlosser, *Fast Food Nation* (Boston: Houghton Mifflin, 2001), pp. 101–102.

No wonder that, by the late 1990s: A. M. Freedman, "Fast Food Chains Play Central Role in Diet of Inner-City Poor," *Wall Street Journal,* December 19, 1990, p. A1.

113 "We knew that kids would want . . .": Interview with Robert Bernstein.

The effort was so important that: Scott Hume, "Research Ignores Preteens: Big Mac Exec," *Advertising Age,* March 17, 1986, p. 28.

114 Pizza Hut changed: "Pizza Hut Targets Kids in Latest TV Push," *Advertising Age,* May 11, 1992, p. 4.

As a team of Columbia University researchers: Emily DeNitto, "Fast-Food Ads Come Under Fire," *Marketing News,* February 14, 1994, p. S14; for an outstanding compendium of such studies, see the Web site for the Center for Science in the Public Interest, the leading advocacy group on the issue, at www.cspinet.org.

115 But in 2001 a group of epidemiologists from the University of Minnesota: S. A. French, M. Story, *et al.,* "Fast food restaurant use among adolescents: associations with nutrient intake, food choices and behavioral and psychosocial variables," *International Journal of Obesity,* v. 25, 2001, pp. 1823–1833.
"Fast food restaurant use was positively associated": *Ibid.,* p. 1823.
Worse, they added, "eating habits established in adolescence . . .": *Ibid.,* p. 1832.
the anthropologist Deborah Crooks: Interview with Deborah Crooks; also, Deborah Crooks, "Child growth and nutritional status in a high-poverty community in eastern Kentucky," *American Journal of Physical Anthropology,* v. 109, 1999, pp. 129–142.

116 "height and weight are cumulative measures . . .": *Ibid.,* p. 138.
"Given that as a nation . . .": *Ibid.,* p. 141.

117 "In heterogeneous and affluent . . .": Peter J. Brown and Vicki K. Bentley-Condit, "Culture, Evolution, and Obesity," *Handbook of Obesity,* ed. George Bray, Claude Bouchard, and W. P. T. James (New York: Marcel Dekker, 1998), p. 149.
"In white girls . . .": Kimm *et al.,* "Race, socioeconomic status . . . ," p. 271. See also T. J. Parsons, C. Power, *et al.,* "Childhood predictors of adult obesity: a systematic review," *International Journal of Obesity,* v. 23, supp. 8, November 1999, pp. s1–s71. Although the inverse correlation is strongest among women in developed nations, it cuts across a surprising range of gender, ethnic, and racial groups as well. The inverse relationship can also extend across generations, even when the individual occupies a higher social address. See Albert J. Strunkard, "Socioeconomic Status and Obesity," in *The Origins and Consequences of Obesity* (New York: Wiley, 1996), pp. 174–206.
"The increase in the prevalence . . .": Seidell and Rissanden, "Worldwide Prevalence of Obesity," in *The Origins and Consequences of Obesity,* p. 87.
"Believe me, it isn't easy . . .": Richard Klein, *Eat Fat* (New York: Vintage, 1996), p. 17.
"With the sort of irony . . .": *Ibid.,* p. 243.

118 Looking for evidence that black girls: See Christian Lawrence and Mark Thelan, "Body image, dieting, and self-concept: their relation in African-American and Caucasian children," *Journal of Clinical Child Psychology,* v. 24, 1995, pp. 41–48.
As *Newsweek* proclaimed: Michelle Ingrassia, "The Body of the Beholder," *Newsweek,* April 24, 1995, pp. 66–67.
"You got to be real fat for me to notice": *Ibid.,* p. 67.

119 "to eliminate a predominantly white Anglo Saxon": M. G. Melnyk and E. Weinstein, "Preventing obesity in black women by targeting adolescents: a literature review," *Journal of the American Dietetic Association,* v. 94, May 1994, pp. 536–540.

After adjusting for respondents' weight: Lawrence B. Rosenfeld, Stephanie C. Stewart, and Heather J. Stinnett, "Preferences for body type and body characteristics associated with attractive and unattractive bodies: Jackson and McGill revisited," *Perceptual and Motor Skills,* v. 89, 1999, pp. 459–470.

"The importance of round buttocks . . .": *Ibid.,* p. 468.

120 "Men and women, regardless of race . . .": *Ibid.,* p. 464.

"although it has been proposed that certain subcultures . . .": R. M. Rebeck, F. M. Cachelin, *et al.,* "Body Size Preferences Across Ethnic Groups: Presented at the Annual Meeting of the North American Association for the Study of Obesity, 2000" (Los Angeles: Department of Psychology, California State University at Los Angeles), p. 2.

A report in the journal *Clinical Pediatrics:* B. A. Sisson, S. M. Franco, *et al.,* "Bodyfat analysis and perception of body image," *Clinical Pediatrics,* v. 36, 1997, pp. 415–418.

121 "That's the big conundrum": Interview with Richard MacKenzie, quoted in Greg Critser, "Let Them Eat Fat," *Harper's,* March 2000, p. 42.

"The number of kids with eating disorders . . .": Interview with Judith Stern, quoted in *Ibid.*

"Social stigma may serve to control obesity . . .": S. Averett and S. Korenman, "Black-white differences in social and economic consequences of obesity," *International Journal of Obesity,* v. 23, 1999, pp. 166–173. For an elaboration on this theme, see K. J. Flynn and M. Fitzgibbon, "Body images and obesity risk among black females: a review of the literature," *Annals of Behavioral Medicine,* v. 20, Winter 1998, pp. 13–24. The authors note: "Body images of black females may contribute to their high risk for obesity by inhibiting motivation for weight control."

122 "Ms. Lopez has a nice big muscled . . .": Quoted in Greg Critser, "The Meridian Candidate," *Worth,* February 1999, p. 122.

"Being a black woman . . .": Erin J. Aubry, "Back Is Beautiful," Salon.com, July 15, 1998.

123 "Compulsive eating in women is a response . . .": Susie Orbach, *Fat Is a Feminist Issue* (New York: Galahad Books, 1997), pp. 33–34, 23, 25.

"Fat is a social disease . . .": *Ibid.,* pp. 22–23.

123 "An early and distinctive psychotherapy of middle class . . .": Joan Jacobs Brumberg, *Fasting Girls* (Cambridge, Massachusetts: Harvard University Press, 1988, rev. 2000), p. 3.

"The association's materials . . .": *Ibid.,* pp. 19–20; see pp. 12–14 for Brumberg's own statistics; for a more recent statistical summation, which puts the rate of anorexia among adolescent and young adult women at .5 to 1 percent, see Susan Zelitch Yanofski, *Obesity and Eating Disorders* (Bethesda, Maryland: National Institute of Diabetes and Digestive and Kidney Diseases, 1997), p. 116.

"a highly specific social address": Brumberg, *Fasting Girls,* p. 13.

124 "can legitimately be called a popular saint": Jennifer Egan, "Power Suffering," *New York Times Magazine,* May 16, 1999, p. 112.

"parents sort of freak out": Interview with James R. Whitehead.

125 There were no effects . . . : J. R. Whitehead and R. C. Ecklund, "Cognitive and Affective Outcomes of Skinfold Caliper Use in Middle School Physical Education: Presentation to 1997 Conference of the American College of Sports Medicine" (Grand Forks, North Dakota: Department of Health and Physical Education, University of North Dakota, 1997).

Similar studies: See, for example, Joseph E. Prusak III, James R. Whitehead, Ronald H. Brinkert, and Robert C. Ecklund, "The Effects of Fitness Testing on Social Physique Anxiety and Physical Self-Perception: Presentation to 2000 Conference of the American Alliance for Health, Physical Education, Recreation and Dance (AAHPERD)" (Grand Forks, North Dakota: Department of Health and Physical Education, University of North Dakota, 2000); and James R. Whitehead and Melissa A. Parker, "Fitness Tests as Opportunities for Cognitive Learning: An Experiment Using Skinfold Testing: 1992 AAHPERD Conference Presentation" (Grand Forks, North Dakota: Department of Health and Physical Education, University of North Dakota, 1992). On a related research question — does dieting cause psychological stress? — see M. L. Klem and M. Y. McGuire, "Psychological symptoms in individuals successful at long-term maintenance of weight loss," *Health Psychology,* v. 17, July 1998, pp. 336–345.

"I don't come to that conclusion lightly": Whitehead interview.

"I am convinced that the drug for treating . . .": Interview with Francine Kaufman.

126 The plant is the largest factory dedicated: Greg Critser, "Your Money and Your Life," *Worth,* March 2000, p. 116.

A recent advertisement for the drug Avandia: See advertising section, *New England Journal of Medicine,* v. 346, March 14, 2002, pp. 875–878.

126 "These days, you've got to be in diabetes": Interview with James Kappel, public relations officer, Eli Lilly and Company. See also Critser, "Let Them Eat Fat," p. 44.

6. What the Extra Calories Do to You

In recent years, the amount of information about the medical consequences of obesity has exploded. Two journals, *Obesity Research* and the *International Journal of Obesity*, remain as the premier organs of the field. In addition, the *Lancet*, the *New England Journal of Medicine*, and the *American Journal of Clinical Nutrition* often publish obesity-related studies. Several lengthy interviews with Dr. Francine Kaufman, head of the children's diabetes clinic at Children's Hospital Los Angeles and president of the American Diabetes Association, helped me understand the real-world implications of those works. The journals *Diabetes* and *Diabetologia* were also important sources on the obesity-diabetes link. A recent book worth every bit of its price for its general wisdom on the subject is Gerald Reaven's *Syndrome X* (New York: Simon & Schuster, 2000).

Data about the connection among fast food, entrepreneurs, and government policy were provided by the Small Business Administration, which performed a special computer tabulation for me to measure the extent of SBA loan guarantees to inner-city fast-food franchisees. In this I was aided by Eric Schlosser's groundbreaking *Fast Food Nation* (Boston: Houghton Mifflin, 2001). In an interview, Robert Bernstein gave me a colorful account of the creation of Happy Meals.

On the subject of "third world peoples living in first world nutritional infrastructures," I was fortunate to have the cooperation of Professor Barry Bogin, whose work on the anthropology of human growth has raised the bar for everyone working in that field; his most recent book, *The Growth of Humanity* (New York: Wiley-Liss, 2001), has become required reading, particularly for anyone involved in nutritional policy-making. The metabolic consequences of fructose, though a relatively new subject, are covered in a number of professional journals, the *American Journal of Clinical Nutrition* chief among them; I was guided through that maze of work by Dr. Scott Connelly, whose recent book, *Body Rx* (New York: Putnam, 2001), takes up the subject and a number of other metabolic issues. The publications and Web site of the Center for Science in the Public Interest also offer substantive work on the subject.

128 "Chocolate iced custard filled" became: *"Durante los últimos 62 años hemos vendido nuestras doughnuts frescas y calientitas,"*

Krispy Kreme promotional flyer, Wendy R. Glickman, public affairs, Great Circle Family Foods, Los Angeles, California.

128 "See," he said, checking his watch: Author interview.

129 "The insulin-resistance gene has protected . . .": Leif C. Groop and Johan G. Eriksson, "The etiology and pathogenesis of non-insulin-dependent diabetes," *Annals of Medicine,* v. 24, 1992, pp. 483–489.

130 "What we are seeing is a mismatch . . .": Interview with Barry Bogin. See also Barry Bogin and James Loucky, "Plasticity, political economy, and physical growth status of Guatemala Maya children living in the United States," *American Journal of Physical Anthropology,* v. 102, 1997, pp. 17–32. For an example of in utero programming theory and its application to fetal nutrition, see K. M. Godfrey and D. J. Barker, "Fetal nutrition and adult disease," *American Journal of Clinical Nutrition,* v. 71, 5 (supp.), 2000, pp. s1344–s1352.
Bogin also notes: Bogin and Loucky, "Plasticity, political economy, and physical growth . . . ," p. 27.

131 Studying fifty-eight pre-pubertal boys: D. J. Hoffman, A. L. Sawaya, *et al.,* "Energy expenditure of stunted and nonstunted boys and girls living in the shantytowns of São Paulo, Brazil," *American Journal of Clinical Nutrition,* v. 72, 2000, pp. 1025–1031.
"the child of obese parents is at increased risk . . .": T. J. Parsons *et al.,* "Childhood predictors of adult obesity," *International Journal of Obesity,* v. 23, supp. 8, 1999, p. s6. For a discussion of childhood obesity tracking into adult obesity, see Nicolas Stettler, "Infant weight gain and childhood overweight status," *Pediatrics,* v. 109, 2002, pp. 194–199.
The current obesity rate for Mexican American children: R. R. Suminski, W. S. Poston, A. S. Jackson, and J. P. Foreyt, "Early identification of Mexican American children who are at risk for becoming obese," *International Journal of Obesity-Related Metabolic Disorders,* v. 23, 1999, pp. 823–829.

132 "And it's one of the first things . . .": Interview with Scott Loren-Selco.
"As endocrinologists, all of us were aware . . .": Interview with Francine Kaufman.

133 "we could see that . . .": *Ibid.*
In 1992, for example, most pediatric diabetes centers: Francine Ratner Kaufman, "Type 2 Diabetes in Children: A New Epidemic," unpublished paper, Department of Endocrinology and Metabolism, Children's Hospital Los Angeles, 2001.

135 "thrifty gene" scholars have even pinpointed: Leif C. Groop and

Tiinamaija Tuomi, "Non-insulin-dependent diabetes mellitus — a collision between thrifty genes and an affluent society," *Annals of Medicine,* v. 29, 1997, pp. 37–53; see also Silva Arslanian and Satish Kalhan, "Correlations between fatty acid and glucose metabolism," *Diabetes,* v. 43, 1994, pp. 908–914.

136 "the more obese you are": Gerald Reaven, *Syndrome X* (New York: Simon & Schuster, 2000), p. 59.

When that happens, according to Victor Zammit: For an outstanding summary of this work see Gail Vines, "Sweet but Deadly," *New Scientist,* September 1, 2001, p. 26; see also A. W. Thorburn, L. H. Storlein, *et al.,* "Fructose-induced in vivo insulin resistance and elevated plasma triglyceride levels in rats," *American Journal of Clinical Nutrition,* v. 49, 1989, pp. 1155–1163.

137 when researchers at the University of Toronto: Vines, "Sweet but Deadly."

Two years ago: John P. Bantle, Susan K. Raatz, *et al.,* "Effects of dietary fructose on plasma lipids in healthy subjects," *American Journal of Clinical Nutrition,* v. 72, 2000, pp. 1128–1134.

To put a point on such observations: C. B. Hollenbeck, "Dietary fructose effects on lipoprotein metabolism and risk for coronary artery disease," *American Journal of Clinical Nutrition,* v. 58, 1993, pp. s800–s809.

The fructose trouble hardly ends there: Y. K. Park and E. A. Yetley, "Intakes and food sources of fructose in the U.S.," *American Journal of Clinical Nutrition,* v. 58, 1993, pp. s737–s747; and Vines, "Sweet but Deadly," p. 29.

138 The theory has its origins in the 1970s, when European: J. Bremer, K. S. Bjerve, *et al.,* "The glycerophosphate acyltransfereses and their function in the metabolism of fatty acids," *Molecular Cell Biochemistry,* v. 12, 1976, pp. 113–125.

The connection with obesity grew when: M. A. McCrory, Paul J. Fuss, *et al.,* "Dietary variety within food groups: association with energy intake and body fatness in men and women," *American Journal of Clinical Nutrition,* v. 69, 1999, pp. 440–447. The study is particularly important for its focus on dietary variety: Does increased, indeed excessive, variety account for the rising rate of obesity, particularly the astounding rise in high-sugar snacks?

139 "Long-term absorption of fructose": P. A. Mayes, "Intermediary metabolism of fructose," *American Journal of Clinical Nutrition,* v. 58, 1993, pp. s754–s765.

By 1995 a farsighted team: J. M. Schwarz, R. A. Neese, *et al.,* "Short-term alterations in carbohydrate energy intake in humans," *Journal of Clinical Investigations,* v. 96, 1995, pp. 2735–2743; for a look at the subject of nutrient partitioning — how the cell "decides" what to burn and what to store, see also O. Ziegler, D. Quilliot, *et al.,* "Macronutrients, fat mass, fatty acid flux and insulin sensitivity," *Diabetes Metabolism,* v. 27, pt. 2, 2001, pp. 261–270; for a look at how high-carbohydrate, high-sugar diets increase the rate of newly synthesized fatty acids and triglycerides, see L. C. Hudgins, "Effect of high carbohydrate feeding on triglyceride and saturated fatty acid synthesis," *Proceedings of the Society of Experimental Biological Medicine,* v. 225, 2000, pp. 178–183.

140 "Consumption of sugar[HFCS]-sweetened drinks": D. S. Ludwig, K. E. Peterson, and S. L. Gortmaker, "Relation between consumption of sugar-sweetened drinks and childhood obesity," *Lancet,* v. 357, 2001, pp. 505–508.

Palm oil's impact on insulin effectiveness: J. M. van Amelsvoort, A. van der Beek, *et al.,* "Dietary influence on the insulin function in the epididymal fat cell of the Wistar rat. I. Effect of type of fat," *Annals of Nutrition and Metabolism,* v. 32, 1988, pp. 138–148; see also J. M. van Amelsvoort *et al.,* "Effects of the type of dietary fatty acid on the insulin receptor function in rat epididymal fat cells," *Annals of Nutrition and Metabolism,* v. 30, 1986, pp. 273–280, which showed that a diet high in sunflower seed oil induced a better response of fat cells to insulin than did a diet high in palm oil.

142 "In contrast to other types of colic . . .": *The Merck Manual of Diagnosis and Therapy* (Whitehouse Station, N.J.: Merck Research Laboratories, 1999), pp. 400–410.

may contract liver steatosis: A. Must and R. S. Strauss, "Risks and consequences of childhood and adolescent obesity," *International Journal of Obesity,* v. 23, supp. 2, pp. s2–s11.

About 40 to 60 percent of adult women: *Ibid.,* p. s4.

Then there are the eyes: *Merck Manual,* p. 168.

143 (A new study shows that structural . . .): Patrick Tounian, Yacine Aggouhn, *et al.,* "Presence of increased stiffness of the common carotid artery and endothelial dysfunction in severely obese children: a prospective study," *Lancet,* v. 358, 2001, pp. 1400–1404.

go something like this: Reaven, *Syndrome X,* pp. 54–55.

144 As the name suggests, this is a brain tumor–like: Must and Strauss, "Risks and consequences . . . ," p. s3.

Then there are the orthopedic problems: *Ibid.*

"The patient is a 14 and one half": Steven R. Boyea and J. Richard

Bowen, "Clinical Case Presentation: Orthopaedic Dept." (Wilmington, Delaware: Alfred I. Du Pont Institute, June 10, 1996), p. 1.

145 The first, Pickwickian syndrome: Must and Strauss, "Risks and consequences . . . ," p. s3.
"Obese children with obstructive sleep apnea . . .": *Ibid.*
Lastly there is the condition known as allergic asthma: *Ibid.* See also T. A. Platts-Mills, M. C. Carter, and P. W. Heymann, "Specific and non-specific obstructive lung disease in childhood: causes of changes in the prevalence of asthma," *Environmental Health Perspectives,* v. 108, supp. 4, 2000, pp. s725–s731; J. A. Castro-Rodriguez, C. J. Holberg, *et al.,* "Increased incidence of asthmalike symptoms in girls who become overweight or obese during school years," *American Journal of Respiratory and Critical Care,* v. 163, 2001, pp. 1344–1349; and P. F. Belamarich, E. Luder, *et al.,* "Do obese inner-city children with asthma have more symptoms than nonobese children with asthma?" *Pediatrics,* v. 106, 2000, pp. 1436–1441; *March of Dimes, Nutrition Today Matters Tomorrow: A Report from the March of Dimes Task Force on Nutrition and Optimal Human Development* (White Plains, N.Y.: March of Dimes, 2002), executive summary, pp. 1–10.

146 In early 2001 the American Cancer Society: Edward Edelson, "Cancer Society Warns on Obesity," *Healthscout Reporter,* January 15, 2001; D. S. Michaud, E. Giovannucci, *et al.,* "Physical activity, obesity, height, and the risk of pancreatic cancer," *Journal of the American Medical Association,* v. 286, 2001, pp. 921–929; J. R. Daling, K. E. Malone, *et al.,* "Relation of body mass index to tumor markers and survival among young women with invasive ductal breast carcinoma," *Cancer,* v. 92, 2001, pp. 720–729; D. M. Purdie and A. C. Green, "Epidemiology of endometrial cancer," *Best Practices of Residential Clinical Obstetrics and Gynaecology,* v. 15, 2001, pp. 341–354.
There are, first and foremost, the premature deaths: D. B. Allison and K. R. Fontaine, "Annual deaths attributable to obesity in the United States," *Journal of the American Medical Association,* v. 282, 1999, pp. 1530–1538.

147 Obesity takes its toll on our daily quality of life: A. M. Wolf and G. A. Colditz, "Current estimates of the economic cost of obesity in the United States," *Obesity Research,* v. 6, 1998, pp. 97–106.
"The economic and personal health costs . . .": *Ibid.*

148 "obesity would account for 132,900 cases of hypertension . . .": G. Oster, J. Edelberg, A. K. O'Sullivan, and D. Thompson, "The clinical

and economic burden of obesity in a managed care setting," *American Journal of Managed Care,* v. 6, 2000, pp. 681–689.

148 "We believe the effect will be like that of secondhand smoke": Interview with James Hill.

149 "We have a long long way to go until . . .": Interview with Gerry Oster, Policy Analysis Inc.

"There's a moment in the Barbara Walters interview . . .": Quoted in Sarah Boxer, "Trash Tropes and Queer Theory: Decoding the Lewinsky Scandal," *New York Times,* August 5, 2001, Week in Review, p. 7.

150 "We got very interested in this area some time ago . . .": Interview with Johannes Hebebrand.

To find out if that were the case: J. Hebebrand, H. Wulftaig, *et al.,* "Epidemic obesity: are genetic factors involved via increased rates of assortative mating?" *International Journal of Obesity,* v. 24, 2000, pp. 345–353.

151 "It is not exactly a straight line": Hebebrand interview.

Yet in this case, recognizing such a dynamic might help prevent: For a discussion about how obese-prone individuals pass on enhanced obesity — in essence a metabolism that defends against weight loss because it has been triggered to do so by weight gain — to subsequent generations, see Barry E. Levin, "The obesity epidemic: metabolic imprinting on genetically susceptible neural circuits," *Obesity Research,* v. 8, 2000, pp. 342–347.

7. What Can Be Done

The discussion of obesity and treatment — both clinical and preventive — generally divides into two categories, that of public health interventions and that of individual medical treatment. An outstanding starting point for those curious about both can be found at the Web site (www.surgeon general.gov) for U.S. Surgeon General David Satcher; the site includes the complete 2002 report *The Surgeon General's Call to Action to Prevent and Decrease Overweight and Obesity,* which does an admirable job of marrying the dual concepts of personal and public responsibility in meeting the challenge. (That both liberals and conservatives took such great umbrage at Satcher's call for all Americans to lose ten pounds says much about how on-spot this report was.) The *Health Professionals Follow-Up Study* and related reports run out of the Harvard School of Public Health are an important source of epidemiological data upon which an increasing number of organizations base their public health interventions. One can read the original studies, with footnotes, as well as a continually updated newsletter, at www.hsph.harvard.edu/hpfs. I was fortunate to have the cooperation of the study's two principal investigators, Walter Willett and Meir Stampfer. To read another important report, *Innovative Approaches to Prevention of Obesity,* and federally funded programs to do so, see www.grants.nih.gov/grants, where the National Institutes of Health tracks such efforts. For evaluations of school-based programs the American Council of School Health offers a number of publications, available at www.ashaweb.org.

At the community level, I interviewed a number of health and medical advocates, many of whom have already put their ideas into fruitful action. Among them were Dr. Robert Trevino, Dr. Francine Kaufman, Marsha MacKenzie, Dan Latham, and several members of the Sacramento Unified School District. Regarding public policy, I interviewed Andrew Hagelshaw at Berkeley's Center for Commercial-Free Public Education, Michael Jacobson at the Center for Science in the Public Interest, Patrick Escobar at the Amateur Athletic Foundation of Los Angeles, and Betty Hennessy of the Los Angeles County Department of Education. To understand more about industry and its response to the issue, I relied heavily on James O. Hill at the University of Colorado, and John Peters at Procter & Gamble.

155 About five years ago: Interview with Robert Trevino; see also R. P. Trevino, R. M. Marshall, D. E. Hale, R. Rodriguez, G. Baker, and J. Gomez, "Diabetes risk factors in low-income Mexican-American children," *Diabetes Care,* v. 22, 1999, pp. 202–207; and Randi Hutter Epstein, "As Diabetes Strikes Younger, Children Get Lessons in Defense," *New York Times,* February 20, 2001, p. D7.
"We scared the hell out of them": Trevino interview.

156 "It's not a gene thing": *Ibid.*
"We didn't believe it was enough . . .": *Ibid.*

157 A year later: R. Trevino, "Bienestar: a diabetes risk-factor prevention program," *Journal of School Health,* v. 68, 1998, p. 62.

158 "clinically significant changes for obese children are rare . . .": T. J. Coates and C. E. Thoresen, "Treating obesity in children and adolescents: a review," *American Journal of Public Health,* v. 68, 1978, pp. 143–151; see also T. N. Robinson, "Behavioural treatment of childhood and adolescent obesity," *International Journal of Obesity,* v. 23, supp. 2, 1999, pp. s52–s57.
By 1994 the general wisdom on the subject: Quoted in Robinson, "Behavioural treatment . . . ," p. s52.
Numerous recent studies — across large numbers of diverse: See, for

example, L. H. Epstein, A. Valoski, *et al.,* "Ten-year follow-up of behavioral, family-based treatment for obese children," *Journal of the
American Medical Association,* v. 264, 1990, pp. 764–770; L. H.
Epstein *et al.,* "Ten-year outcomes of behavioral, family-based treatment for childhood obesity," *Health Psychology,* v. 13, 1994,
pp. 373–383.

159 The cornerstone of his approach . . . the Stoplight Diet: L. H. Epstein
and S. Squires, *The Stoplight Diet for Children: An Eight-Week Program for Parents and Children* (Boston: Little, Brown, 1988).

160 "It is our experience that some patients . . .": Quoted in Robinson,
"Behavioural treatment . . . ," pp. s53–s54.

161 Yet Epstein, unlike a generation of: *Ibid.;* see also Epstein *et al.,*
"Ten-year follow-up . . . ,": and Epstein *et al.,* "Ten-year outcomes . . ."

162 "What's amazing is how uninhibited . . .": Interview with Marsha
MacKenzie.
"We have to start from ground zero": *Ibid.*

163 "That drives the point home . . .": *Ibid.*
The students were able to achieve and sustain: Kelly Brownell and
Frederick Kaye, "A school-based behavior modification, nutrition education, and physical activity program for obese children," *American
Journal of Clinical Nutrition,* v. 35, 1982, pp. 277–283.
"It is interesting that few studies . . .": M. Story, "School-based approaches for preventing and treating obesity," *International Journal
of Obesity,* v. 23, supp. 2, 1999, pp. s43–s51.
A more recent survey, based on in-depth interviews with sixty-one
overweight: Dianne Neumark-Sztainer and Mary Story, "Recommendations from overweight youth regarding school-based weight control programs," *Journal of School Health,* v. 67, 1997, pp. 428–433.

164 In a study by the University of Houston and Baylor College: R.
Suminski *et al.,* "Early identification of Mexican American children
who are at risk for becoming obese," *International Journal of Obesity,* v. 23, August 1999, p. 823.
Researchers from Stanford's Departments of Pediatrics and Medicine: Thomas N. Robinson, "Reducing children's television viewing
to prevent obesity," *Journal of the American Medical Association,* v.
282, 1999, pp. 1561–1567.

165 While not an anticipated outcome, the intervention group also "significantly . . .": *Ibid.,* p. 1564.

166 Whatever the cause, the Stanford researchers concluded: *Ibid.,*
p. 1561.
"The challenge in changing the environment is not to 'go back in

time,' . . .": Quoted in John C. Peters, Holly R. Wyatt, William T. Donahoo, and James O. Hill, "From instinct to intellect: the challenge of maintaining healthy weight in the modern world," *Obesity Reviews*, forthcoming.

167 One of them is Dan Latham: Interview with Dan Latham; see also Greg Critser, "A Get Fit Plan . . . ," *Los Angeles Times*, December 16, 2001, p. M3.

168 "What we found startled us . . .": *Ibid.*

169 "Frankly, it was such a done deal . . .": Interview with Michelle Masoner, board member, Sacramento Unified Schools.

"We looked closely at the contract . . .": Interview with Manny Hernandez, board member, Sacramento Unified Schools.

"We decided that we had to make the health case . . .": Masoner interview.

170 "The kids were telling us they loved it": Hernandez interview.

The most common comes in the form of "sponsored educational materials": Interview with Andrew Hagelshaw, Center for Commercial-Free Public Education.

"We are seeing hundreds of groups . . .": *Ibid.*

171 A few weeks later, the army: Reuters News Service, "Obesity Is Increasing in the Military," *Los Angeles Times*, November 11, 2001, p. A35.

172 Average PE class size: See Critser, "A Get Fit Plan . . ."; Duke Helfand, "State Youths Flunk Fitness Exam," *Los Angeles Times*, December 11, 2001, p. B1; Betty Hennessy and John Martois, "A Comparison of Student Reading Scores on the SAT-9 and Achievement of Healthy Fitness Zones on the Fitnessgram," paper presented to annual conference of the Society of State Directors for Health, Physical Education, and Dance, Orlando, Florida, March 19, 2000, available through Los Angeles Department of Education.

173 Instead, "we might start thinking of them as unified . . .": Interview with Walter Willett; see also his *Eat, Drink and Be Healthy* (New York: Simon & Schuster, 2001).

"And when I say exercise": Willett interview.

Of these, the most controversial is the "fat tax": Michael Jacobson and Kelly Brownell, "Small taxes on soft drinks and snack foods to promote health," *American Journal of Public Health*, v. 90, 2000, pp. 854–857.

A TV and radio campaign in Clarksburg: *Ibid.*, p. 855.

174 "But it is always held up by the basic marketing . . .": Interview with John Peters.

175 For we need only look to previous eras: See Emmett Rice, *A Brief History of Physical Education* (New York: A. S. Barnes, 1926).
As one of its founders, Dr. Charles Beck: Quoted in *Ibid.,* p. 153.

176 "eternal, cold and cursed heavy rain": Dante Alighieri, *The Divine Comedy: Inferno,* ed. and trans. Robert Durling (New York: Oxford, 1996), p. 101.
"languish in the black slime": *Ibid.,* p. 119.

INDEX